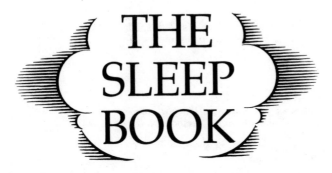

THE SLEEP BOOK

Understanding and Preventing Sleep Problems in People Over 50

ERNEST HARTMANN, M.D.

An AARP Book
published by
American Association of Retired Persons, Washington, D.C.
Scott, Foresman and Company, Lifelong Learning Division,
Glenview, Illinois

Figures 4–14 on pages 24, 26, 28, 29, 30, 31, 33, 34, and 35 adapted from *Electroencephalography (EEG) of Human Sleep: Clinical Applications* by Williams, Karacan, and Hursch. Copyright © 1974 by John Wiley & Sons, Inc. Reprinted by permission.

Appendix A adapted from "Outline of Diagnostic Classification of Sleep and Arousal Disorders" from *Sleep*, vol. 2, no. 1. Copyright © 1979 Raven Press, New York. Reprinted by permission.

Sleep disorders centers and sleep disorders specialists from *Roster of Centers*, January 1, 1987, Association of Sleep Disorders Centers. Reprinted by permission.

Library of Congress Cataloging-in-Publication Data

Hartmann, Ernest.
    The sleep book.

    Includes index.
    1. Sleep disorders—Popular works. 2. Sleep disorders—Age factors. 3. Insomnia—Popular works. 4. Aged—Diseases—Popular works. I. Title.
RC547.H37 1987   618.97′6849   87–4479
ISBN 0-673-24825-9 (Scott Foresman)

AARP Books is an educational and public service project of the American Association of Retired Persons, which, with a membership of more than 24 million, is the largest association of persons fifty and over in the world today. Founded in 1958, AARP provides older Americans with a wide range of membership programs and services, including legislative representation at both federal and state levels. For further information about additional association activities, write to AARP, 1909 K Street, N.W., Washington, DC 20049.

Other Books by Ernest Hartmann
The Biology of Dreaming
Adolescents in a Mental Hospital
The Functions of Sleep
The Sleeping Pill
The Nightmare: The Psychology and Biology of
    Terrifying Dreams
Sleep and Dreaming (editor)

Contents

v

Introduction

We spend our lives in two basic states—wakefulness and sleep. Those of us who live to be a hundred will have spent perhaps thirty years in the state of sleep. Yet sleep has remained a blank in our medical and scientific awareness until a few decades ago. Only recently have researchers learned the mechanics of sleep and, among other findings, discovered how much can go wrong within this state.

Sleep and sleep disorders are of special interest to older persons. So many aspects of sleep—number of awakenings, total time spent awake, and time spent in the various sleep stages—change dramatically with age, and the kind of problems that can occur in our sleep-wake patterns also change dramatically with age.

When we talk about sleep disorders, we are not talking about a rare illness that afflicts an occasional unfortunate person. In any one year, 20 to 30 percent of the United States population complain of some form of sleep problem or sleep disorder. Almost all of us have a sleep problem at some point or another during our lives whether with daytime sleepiness or difficulty sleeping at night. The problems, however, are not always serious ones that need immediate expert attention.

I am a physician, a sleep disorders specialist, as well as a psychiatrist. I have treated, studied, and interviewed at least a thousand people with a variety of sleep-related complaints. I am also director of a sleep disorders center associated with Tufts University School of Medicine at the Newton-Wellesley Hospital. A sleep disorders center is a place at which very careful and detailed examinations of sleep patterns can be done, making use of all-night recordings as well as daytime studies to try to pinpoint the exact cause and the best treatment for the most serious sleep problems.

The majority of people with sleep problems do not require the services of a sleep disorders center. If you have a problem with your sleep, there are a number of things you can do for yourself. In the following chapters, I shall try to help you understand normal sleep as well as the changes that occur in normal sleep as we get older. I'll try to help you decide whether any sleep problem you or a loved one may have is serious, or whether it is simply part of everyday life. I shall try to help you figure out whether a serious problem is one that you can deal with yourself (and surprisingly often this is the case), is one that needs the help of your physician, or is a problem that may require further help from a sleep disorders specialist or a sleep disorders center.

◄ 1 ►

Sleep Problems and Disorders in Older Persons

"Someone's attacking me in my sleep." Hannah, fifty-six, says she has been in good health for most of her life. She comes to see me complaining that for about six weeks she has had very strange and frightening nightmares. They involve wars, with a lot of blood and gore; in some she is chased or attacked, or cut to pieces.

For the last few weeks she has not wanted to go to bed because these nightmares and dreams are so disturbing. *All* of her dreams have, in fact, become more vivid and complicated than they were. She used to remember only an occasional vague dream; now she dreams every night—"all sorts of crazy things, horrible things, sometimes nightmares." She knows that severe nightmares sometimes occur at times of stress, but she believes she has no particular problems and feels fine except for the nightmares.

She is a lively and talkative woman, eager to tell me at great length about her family and her part-time job. It

3

is hard for me to get a word in edgewise. But she certainly convinces me that she is not especially anxious and is not about to break down. Nor does she seem at all depressed. There appears to be nothing going on psychologically that would produce this change in sleep and these severe nightmares.

In her case, obtaining a careful medical history leads to the solution to her problems. She assures me she is in good health. She has a physical exam and checkup once a year, just as she has been told she should. She stopped smoking many years ago, drinks a glass of wine several times a week, and says this hasn't changed recently; it couldn't be bothering her. She has had no psychiatric or neurological illness. In fact, she is absolutely well except for a mild elevation in blood pressure, which her internist has been treating "with some sort of pills" for years.

It is only when I ask her in detail about the blood pressure medication that she recalls that at her last yearly physical her internist suggested changing to a different, slightly stronger medication for her high blood pressure. She is now taking propranolol, an effective antihypertensive, also known as a beta-adrenergic blocker. It appears that Hannah's vivid dreams and nightmares began within a week after she changed blood pressure medication. I have seen a number of middle-aged people who have almost exactly this problem, changes in sleep and sometimes very disturbing nightmares, when they start taking propranolol and related drugs.

Hannah was helped simply by changing to another medication for her high blood pressure. She was quite right that there was nothing psychologically wrong and that her life was otherwise going well.

"I wake up, and I can't move." Angela is embarrassed to be seeing a doctor about her problems. She comes mainly because her husband and her sister have

been urging her off and on for years to find out whether there is something wrong.

"Basically, I feel a little silly being here because there's nothing wrong with my sleep. I've always slept pretty well. I fall asleep right away, then maybe wake once or twice during the night—but never enough to bother me. The problem is more in the morning. The problem is kind of funny. I wake up paralyzed, so I can't move. This goes on for a few minutes sometimes, and I think perhaps I'll die from not being able to breathe, but I seem to arouse myself out of it okay. Also, my husband says to tell you I have been kind of sleepy in the daytime for years. I don't mean I'm sleepy all day, but I have these times when I just can't stay awake, and I just have to lie down and take a nap."

It appears that Angela, now fifty-two, has suffered from this pattern of sleepiness in the daytime for a long time—at least twenty years, maybe longer—but has never wanted to make much of an issue of it. She is very shy and does not like to go to doctors. She went to see a doctor years ago, and, in fact, she now recalls that the doctor told her she might have a neurological problem and recommended she go to a specialist. However, she hasn't followed that advice. She has simply adapted to the problem, living a quiet life with her husband, working part-time in the stacks of a library. She reasons, "Some people are just more sleepy than others. I guess some of us need naps in the daytime." Her supervisors, too, know she is prone to taking occasional naps at her workplace but are not especially disturbed by it. So she has not gotten further help, even though it seems that this daytime sleep disrupts her life considerably. Only when she began to have the episodes of paralysis did she finally allow herself to be talked into seeing a specialist.

In Angela's case, daytime recordings in a sleep disorders center—recordings known as a Multiple Sleep Latency Test—allowed us to establish very quickly that she suffered from a recognized disorder called narcolepsy, which accounted for her daytime sleep attacks as well as her morning sleep paralysis. She was treated with medication and careful scheduling of her naps. With these treatments, she suddenly found she had a great deal more energy than before. She began to travel with her husband, take some courses, and think about finding a new and more challenging job.

"I just can't get to sleep." Daniel comes to see me complaining of severe difficulty in falling asleep. He goes to bed at ten or eleven at night and lies for hours without getting to sleep. When he finally does fall asleep, he wakes up at four or five in the morning and tries unsuccessfully to fall back to sleep.

Daniel has no definite medical problems that could account for his sleep disorder. He is an obviously intelligent sixty-seven-year-old man who has been active and cheerful most of his life. Nothing obviously upsetting has happened to him recently. He has a wife and two children and retired two years ago from a good job in an engineering firm. He was busy and active throughout his working life, with very few illnesses and no sleep problems whatever.

He complains that in the past year his sleep problem has become worse and worse and does not respond to medication. He has seen three different doctors, taken sleeping pills, and also tried alcohol at night because a friend told him that a good shot of brandy was what he needed. None of this has helped much; in fact, he feels he is getting worse. The sparkle he usually has in his eyes goes out when he talks about his sleep problem. He says things like, "After all, I have had a good life, and maybe this is just the beginning of the end."

I talk to Daniel about what he has been doing since he retired. It turns out that he meant to continue working part-time consulting with another company but that this did not work out, and he quit. The first year he enjoyed not having much to do. He planned to go on several long trips with his wife. However, she had recently developed an arthritic condition that required frequent medical treatments, so they ended up staying home. Daniel's life, in recent months, has consisted of sitting in a chair watching TV or reading a book for most of the day. Sometimes he feels bored and takes a walk around the block. At times he has a drink by himself or with his wife; it helps pass the time.

When I speak to his wife (an essential part of the evaluation), she confirms that Daniel spends a good deal of time in front of the TV. She tells me that he seems bored and sometimes dozes off for half an hour or an hour at a time.

Putting all this together, it appeared that there was nothing specifically wrong with Daniel's sleep, but there was obviously something unfortunate about the way he was running his life. Watching TV all day can be a depressing way for an intelligent person who has always been active before to spend time. Daniel, in fact, appeared to be obtaining a fair amount of sleep in the daytime while watching TV, so, of course, he was not sleepy when he went to bed at 10:00 P.M. Furthermore, neither his body nor his mind was working much during the day, and for this reason, he did not develop the tiredness one normally feels in the evening and that he used to feel when he was more active.

In this situation, the treatment that Daniel was using could only make his condition worse. Alcohol does indeed have a sedative effect—it knocks you out, but you then tend to wake up much earlier than usual, sometimes after two or three hours. So the alcohol could actually have been contributing to his early morning awakenings. Sleeping pills also may have been making things worse. Most currently used sleeping medication remains in the body a long time—an especially long time in older persons. Thus, when Daniel took the sleeping pills, they may well have contributed to his feeling drowsy in the daytime and may have made it even more likely for him to doze off in front of the TV set. Even without sleeping pills, few people can watch hours of daytime television without becoming sleepy. Thus, the last thing Daniel needed was something to make him more sleepy. He was already leading an overly "sleepy" life since his retirement. What he needed was to become more active—if possible more active both mentally and physically. I talked this over with Daniel and his wife.

When I last saw Daniel, he was exploring a number of possibilities. He was trying to play tennis again, which he hadn't done for years. He first thought this was a crazy idea—how could a sixty-seven-year-old man get back into a tough game like tennis? He said, however, that he had tried it and liked it, and his game was gradually improving. He was also starting in a tentative way to use his engineering and managerial skills. He was giving talks about engineering to interested high-school students and had done some tutoring in his field. He and his wife had jointly decided to do volunteer work at a local hospital, and they had also decided to do the traveling they had kept putting off. They found that once they made up their minds, it was not that difficult to arrange for periodic medical check-ups and even arthritis treatments along their route. When I spoke with Daniel on the phone recently, he seemed a great deal more cheerful and alert. He didn't even mention his sleep problem until I asked him about it; at this point it had lessened considerably and become only a minor detail in his busy life.

"I fell asleep in the middle of a conference with my most important client." The case of Wilcott, a successful lawyer of fifty-nine, is quite different from Daniel's situation. Wilcott claims he sleeps well at night but is worried about increasing tiredness and falling asleep in the daytime. A sharp, alert attorney, famed for his wit as well as for his legal acumen, he has begun to doze at times during the day even though he leads an active professional and social life. He first began to nod off

every day in front of the TV set after dinner, which his family attributed to overwork. Soon he was falling asleep at dinner parties, and during the past year, he has nodded off during important conferences in his law office as well. People have asked him whether he is especially tired or whether he has lost a lot of sleep, and he says no, that he sleeps a lot at night and adds, "Perhaps I'm just getting old." His colleagues and family are quite concerned because he is not only falling asleep more often but seems to be more and more forgetful, and it is obvious that he will soon be unable to continue his work.

A physical examination by his doctor demonstrates nothing unusual. The doctor tells him he is in good health except that his blood pressure is a bit on the high side and he needs to lose a few pounds.

Wilcott's wife contributes an important piece of the puzzle. She confirms his story that he indeed sleeps a long time at night. However, she disagrees with him when he says he sleeps well. From her observations, his sleep is fitful and interrupted. She has not been able to observe him as much as she did in the past; his loud snoring and his fitful sleep have made it impossible for her to obtain any rest at night, so she has moved into the room next door. She can only report what she hears through the walls. Nonetheless, she can say that she hears loud, intermittent snoring during the night, and she sometimes goes in and finds him gasping, rolling over, and even sitting up on the edge of the bed without apparently waking up. When she asks him about it in the morning, he is unaware that anything unusual happened during the night. When pressed, he admits that when he gets up in the morning, he often has a headache and feels poorly rested. However, he shrugs this off: "I'm not one to complain. I spend over eight hours asleep, so I must be okay."

A careful evaluation of Wilcott's situation and an all-night recording of his sleep revealed a condition known as obstructive sleep apnea, which was quite severe in his case. He indeed snored heavily during the night, and a recording showed that he stopped breathing approximately 150 times in the course of a night. He would then arouse himself, take a few breaths, go back to sleep, and restart this cycle. This resulted in a lowered oxygen level in his blood and produced a situation in which he was spending eight hours in bed but getting very little good sleep.

There are a number of treatments that can help in sleep apnea, and these will be discussed further in chapter 7. In Wilcott's case, treatments involved a strict diet to produce weight loss, a method of keeping him from sleeping in certain positions, and a medication, protriptyline. Wilcott is still under treatment but is already greatly improved. He is regaining his old reputation as a brilliant attorney, and he has completely given up his notion that he must just be getting old.

The cases presented here represent only a few of the many sleep problems and disorders that affect older persons. What they show is that sleep is a complex state affecting the body and the mind in numerous ways. Current research into the nature of sleep, modern diagnostic procedures including the use of sleep laboratories, and new methods of classifying disorders can determine whether an individual has a sleep problem that needs treatment.

Treatment for sleep disorders may involve a simple change in the sleep environment or a change of schedule or activity level. It can involve medication—often discontinuing or reducing a medication, or alcohol; at other times taking a new medication aimed at a specific disorder. It can involve counseling or psychotherapy. And, at times, it can involve surgery or other treatment for a serious medical problem.

You can solve some problems yourself; others require professional help. It is important to learn the difference.

◀ 2 ▶

Sleep—A Different
Organization of Life

In Greek mythology, Sleep was the younger sister of Death, and for a long time scientists and doctors considered sleep a kind of lesser form of death. Textbooks are full of diagrams showing a continuum of active wakefulness to sedation to sleep to anesthesia to coma to death; and, unfortunately, many of the "sleeping medications" developed over the years have actions that reflect such a continuum. They produce sedation in small doses, sleep in larger doses, and eventually coma and death in still larger doses.

We have known intuitively for centuries that sleep is important for us. Shakespeare called sleep "Chief nourisher in life's feast," and he also spoke of "Sleep that knits up the ravell'd sleave of care." I believe that Shakespeare was right on both counts. Sleep *is* nourishment; it allows us to rebuild our bodies and brains. In addition, it serves a function related to memory and learning; sleep helps us make connections between re-

11

cent and old memories and helps us "tie up loose ends."

Considering that we spend close to one-third of our lives in sleep, it is amazing that sleep has been seriously studied for only the last thirty years or so. We could say that as scientists we knew almost nothing about sleep until the 1950s. In the past twenty-five years, during which I have been doing research on sleep, a huge amount of information has been collected not only about sleep itself but also about numerous sleep disorders.

WHAT SLEEP IS

Now that we are learning more about the way we sleep, we know that sleep is not half way to death but rather a state we all experience—a state apparently necessary for restoration (though we are still exploring in what ways) and a state characterized not by quiescence or absence of activity but by a very different organization of our bodies and brains. A great deal is happening during sleep. For instance, in our dreams we are conscious; we see and often hear, feel, and experience things, but it is so different from the way we do things when we are awake. We live a different life, as it were, in our dreams. We are using the same brain, the same equipment, as during waking consciousness, but its activity is organized in a different manner.

The body itself is not inactive but simply differently organized during sleep. For instance, our delicately tuned breathing apparatus is something we are not usually even aware of. It breathes for us while we are doing something else. But when we analyze it in detail, it turns out that each breath depends on impulses that are sent out from the brain stem to the diaphragm and the chest initiating inspiration, and others that are sent out for expiration. At the same time, impulses are sent to the muscles in the back of our throat to ensure that the airway is open. Certain sensors tell us that we have too little oxygen or too much carbon dioxide in our blood, that the air passages are not fully open, and so on. It turns out that all these delicate mechanisms are organized differently during sleep and during wakefulness. (Many people who breathe entirely normally when they are awake have problems with breathing while they are asleep.)

Although we know that sleep is a whole state of its own—actually two different states—during which a great deal is happening, scientists have not come up with a perfect definition of sleep. It's one of those things that we all seem to know about but find hard to define. The best definition I can come up with is that sleep is a behavioral state, a regularly recurrent normal behavioral state, characterized by relative quiescence and a great increase in response threshold to the environment; that is, it takes a louder noise or greater stimulation to produce any reaction in a sleeping person than in one who is awake. This is not far from our commonsense impression of sleep—that the sleeper is just lying there and doesn't answer when spoken to.

We now know that this behavioral state is also associated with a biological state, a state of the brain, characterized by decreased activity in some areas of the brain and increased activity in certain other areas. However, the basic definition is still the behavioral one. It is only by studying people and animals in what we know as the behavioral state of sleep that we have been able to determine the biological aspects of sleep.

A NIGHT OF SLEEP

As you begin to fall asleep, you undergo some changes that anyone can observe. Your body moves less, your muscles become relaxed, and your breathing gradually slows down and becomes more regular; there's not much more than that. If you have the patience to watch someone all night though, you notice that sleep is not entirely quiet. The sleeper will move and roll over a number of times during the night; most people—even those who think they sleep in the same position all night—actually change positions about thirty times. If you watch carefully, you will also note periods during which the sleeper's eyes move under the eyelids and when breathing becomes somewhat irregular.

The modern sleep laboratory can help us get further information. By now, many thousands of people have spent one or more nights in a sleep laboratory, and so we can describe in greater detail what happens when someone spends a night sleeping.

First, during sleep onset, breathing and pulse slow down slightly. There are usually a few body movements and sometimes slow movements of the eyes. During this time, the brain waves, the rhythmic electrical activity produced by the brain, undergo a number of changes. Recordings on an electroencephalogram (EEG) show that the mixture of ten-per-second activity (alpha waves) and high-frequency waves that characterizes wakefulness gradually gives way to a pattern of mixed low-voltage activity known as stage 1 sleep—a transitional state. This is followed by a state characterized by sleep spindles—groups of fast waves, thirteen or fifteen per second, which are basically seen only during sleep—and certain spiking waves known as K-complexes. These spindles and K-complexes characterize what we call stage 2 of sleep. Stage 2 is the first stage that everyone recognizes as "definite" sleep.

In the next few minutes in a healthy sleeper, the EEG activity slows down a bit so that there are more and more slow waves. (Slow waves, or delta waves, have a frequency of one-half to four per second.) We somewhat arbitrarily refer to this period as stage 3 of sleep, when at least 20 percent of the record is taken up by slow waves, and then stage 4 of sleep, when at least 50 percent of the record is taken up by slow waves (see figure 1).

Wakefulness

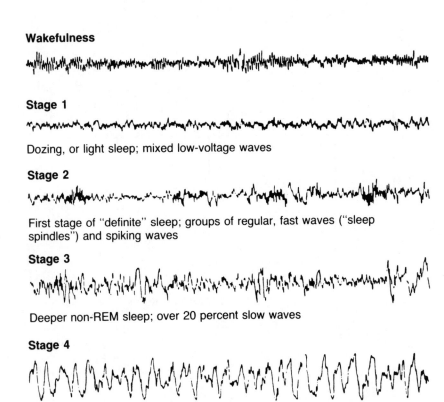

Stage 1

Dozing, or light sleep; mixed low-voltage waves

Stage 2

First stage of "definite" sleep; groups of regular, fast waves ("sleep spindles") and spiking waves

Stage 3

Deeper non-REM sleep; over 20 percent slow waves

Stage 4

Deepest, non-REM sleep; over 50 percent slow waves

Figure 1. Brain-wave patterns during wakefulness and sleep

Adapted from *The Biology of Dreaming* by Ernest Hartmann. Copyright © 1967 by Charles C. Thomas, Publisher, Springfield Illinois. Reprinted by permission.

This progression of sleep stages was discovered in the 1930s; it was assumed that a good night of sleep involved the transition from wakefulness to deep, slow-wave sleep (stage 4 sleep) and then a return to wakefulness. However, the work of recent decades, starting with the studies of Eugene Aserinsky and Nathaniel Kleitman in the 1950s, shows that sleep does not consist of a change from wakefulness to stage 4 to

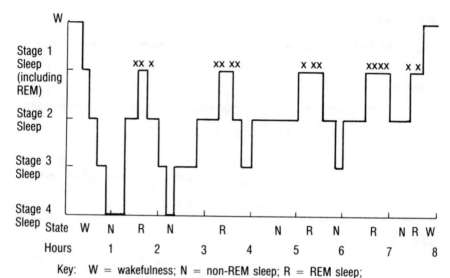

Key: W = wakefulness; N = non-REM sleep; R = REM sleep;
      x = presence and approximate spacing of rapid eye movements

Figure 2. Stages of sleep in a young adult

wakefulness but rather of a number of regular cycles (see figure 2).

What happens is that the sleeper, after one to two hours of stage 2, stage 3, and stage 4 sleep, seems to have a lightening of sleep; there are a few body movements, and the EEG record resembles stage 1 sleep, the lightest stage. At this same time, a number of other changes occur: the eyes begin to move together, sometimes quite rapidly, and the person enters a state known as rapid-eye-movement sleep, or REM sleep. Everything changes somewhat during this time: respiration becomes somewhat faster and definitely more irregular; the same is true of pulse and blood pressure.

During these REM periods, which recur several times during the night, there is an increased activity in many body systems. Everything is slightly aroused, though the sleeper continues sleeping. For instance, men usually have partial or full erections during these periods. Women have some genital changes involving increases in blood flow to the genitals. Furthermore, if one is awakened during these periods, one can usually, but not always, report a dream. For this reason, these periods are known not only as REM sleep, but also as *dreaming sleep*, or as *desynchronized sleep* (D-sleep), since the EEG pattern is irregular, or desynchronized. Still another name for these periods is *paradoxical sleep*. The paradox is that the record looks as though the person is sleeping very lightly, but it is actually quite difficult to arouse the person from this state, so it is light sleep in some ways and deep sleep in others.

Various studies report that from 50 to over 90 percent of the time, sleepers can describe dreams after awakenings from REM sleep. Dreams are sometimes reported from other parts of the night, too, but they are less frequent and less dramatic. The kind of long, complicated, vivid, emotional dream with unusual or bizarre content that we remember later and tell people about seems always to come from REM sleep; "dreaming sleep" is an appropriate name for this state.

These periods of REM sleep, or D-sleep, occur four or five times during a typical night. The pattern shown repeatedly over thousands of recordings is depicted in simplified form in figure 2, and the characteristics are amazingly regular. Reasonably healthy adults, whether they consider themselves wonderfully deep sleepers or light sleepers, whether they remember dreams or do not remember them, go through this same pattern with alternations between non-REM sleep and REM sleep approximately every ninety or one hundred minutes during the night. REM periods increase in length as the night progresses and take up a total of perhaps one-fourth of a night, while non-REM sleep (stages 2, 3, and 4) takes up the other three-fourths of the night.

The two states of sleep—non-REM sleep and REM sleep—are found in all human sleepers and in just about all mammals as well.

SLEEP IN ANIMALS

Owners of young cats and dogs know that their pets have several states of sleep, including times when the pets move their eyes and paws and appear to be dreaming. In fact, we can show by observations and recordings that all mammals have distinct states of sleep very similar to those of human sleep. With only one known exception, all mammals have two separate states of sleep—non-REM sleep and REM sleep. The pattern is not always the same, of course. Mammals do not as a rule spend seven or eight hours asleep in one solid block, as most adult humans do. They may catnap, "dognap," or "mousenap," or have their own characteristic patterns, but when they are asleep, we can record things very similar to what we record in humans, including REM and non-REM sleep.

Mammals that have REM and non-REM sleep all have a cyclic alternation between the two states. The length of this cycle is ninety minutes in humans but varies with the species. Sleep studies on the elephant demonstrate that elephants have REM and non-REM sleep; in fact, they have a cycle longer than that in humans. This corresponds with the fact that most of the body cycles, such as the pulse cycle (the length of a heartbeat) and the respiratory cycle, are longer in large animals such as the elephant and shorter in small animals. Figure 3 shows that the REM/Non-REM cycle differs across species exactly as do other better-known body cycles. Another characteristic pattern is that young mammals always sleep more than adults. Both total sleep time and REM time are high at birth and decrease with age.

With regard to dreams in animals, there are many unanswered questions. The way we tell whether people are dreaming is to wake them up and ask them; we cannot do this with animals. However, since REM sleep in animals involves activation of the same parts of the brain as in humans, including the visual cortex, one can

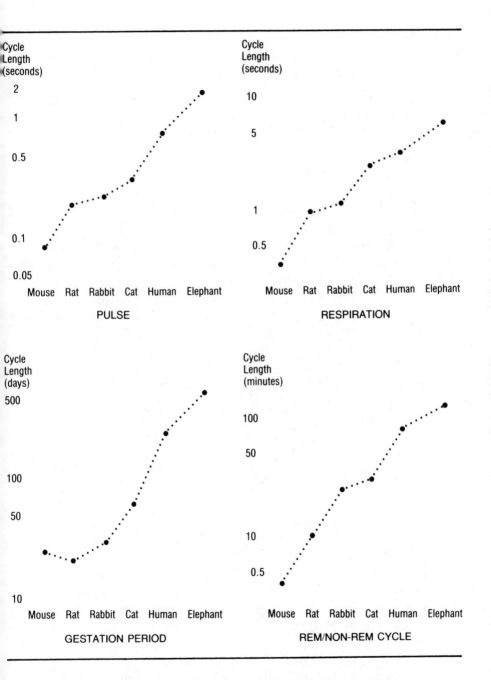

Figure 3. These mammals follow a similar pattern in the four biological cycles shown.

Adapted from *The Biology of Dreaming* by Ernest Hartmann. Copyright © 1967 by Charles C. Thomas, Publisher, Springfield Illinois. Reprinted by permission.

surmise that animals dream. Also, animals do have eye movements, and one can sometimes see young animals running or playing in their sleep during REM periods.

HOW MUCH SLEEP WE NEED

For a time, some serious researchers felt that sleep was a kind of old habit, a behavioral appendix, which we still had in our bodies but did not really require. However, there is not much evidence for this view. Some colleagues and I did a number of studies on sleep requirements and tried hard to find people with a low sleep requirement—people who could get along with less than three or four hours of sleep in twenty-four hours or with no sleep at all. Everyone has a friend who supposedly gets along on almost no sleep, but the story never seems to hold up under close scrutiny. We had fairly strict requirements—we asked people to keep sleep logs for several weeks, we made sleep recordings, and so on. Basically we could find and study in detail no one who regularly slept less than four hours per night. (In these studies, we were not considering people with sleep disorders or severe insomnia but rather people who had unusual but satisfactory patterns of sleep—people who seemed to *require* different amounts.)

We did find, however, that there was considerable variation. There were some who got along fine on five or six hours of sleep per night. (These were people who slept only five or six hours even on Sundays; they did not have to "catch up.") We also found that there were people who required nine or ten hours of sleep and did not feel comfortable unless they obtained this amount. Thus, we believe there is such a thing as sleep requirement, but not everyone needs eight hours of sleep. Statistics suggest that sleep requirements vary from five hours to ten hours in the normal population, with the average at seven to seven-and-a-half hours.

WHAT HAPPENS IF WE DON'T SLEEP

A great many studies of sleep deprivation in animals and humans have been conducted. Sleep deprivation produces characteristic changes in the nervous system—basically activation of the autonomic nervous system along with certain changes (slowed patterns) in brain activity. One can also show changes in behavior and in performance on certain tests, though here the surprising finding has been that a young adult human in good shape performs quite well after two, three, or four nights without any sleep, at least if the performance involves short, intense activity, such as playing Ping-Pong, using pinball machines, or doing arithmetic problems.

The effects of sleep deprivation really show up only when a long, dull task is being performed, such as watching a radar screen and having to respond whenever a certain signal comes up. These findings, of course, are important, since long, dull tasks such as watching radar screens and instrument panels are exactly what our air traffic controllers and pilots have to do occasionally (but we hope not often) with insufficient sleep.

Despite the fact that young adults can function relatively well on many tests when they have missed a couple of nights of sleep, we all know that losing sleep makes us feel miserable. We have some kind of subjective feeling that is more sensitive to sleep loss than the objective tests. And if we wish, we can measure this subjective state by asking people to fill out questionnaires as to how they feel.

It is, of course, easy to study total sleep deprivation for a day or two but much harder to study the effects of small amounts of sleep loss over a long period. It is the study of this kind of partial sleep deprivation that is important in understanding and trying to help people with various kinds of insomnia and conditions that interfere with sleep.

WHY WE SLEEP

There is still no universal agreement on why we sleep. A great deal of evidence exists for the view that sleep does have a function; in fact sleep has two related functions, one for each of the two related states of sleep—non-REM and REM sleep.

Non-REM sleep appears to be required for a basic function involving synthesis of macromolecules (proteins, RNA, and so on) in the body and especially in the brain—a basic restorative function that precedes and lays the groundwork for the REM-sleep function. REM sleep then has a function relating to memory and learning. It is involved in tying up loose ends; smoothing things out emotionally; and connecting recent material with old pathways, wishes, and fears. REM sleep may also be involved in restoring the function of the cortex and certain brain pathways that are involved in attention, learning, and other daytime functions.

Most researchers now accept the fact that sleep has one and perhaps two such biological functions; however, there is no complete agreement, nor are the functions totally understood.

Although we cannot yet specify exactly why we need sleep, it appears that we do need it, and we need it all through our lives. Sleep does change with age, however.

◀ 3 ▶

Changes in Sleep Patterns
with Age

As you get older, you will probably notice that your sleep changes a bit. For some, the changes are quite dramatic; for others, they are more subtle. And an occasional person claims not to notice any change.

The most common change is that we wake up more often during the night and spend more time awake during the night; most people report at least some change in this regard. For some, there is a decrease in sleep requirement; someone who used to need seven hours of sleep per night gets along on six, but this is not true of everyone. In fact, some people seem to need more sleep as they get older.

In any case, some changes in sleep patterns almost always occur; this is hardly surprising because everything changes to some extent as we get older. If you know what is normal and expectable at your age, you will be in a better position to decide whether your particular sleep pattern is something to worry about.

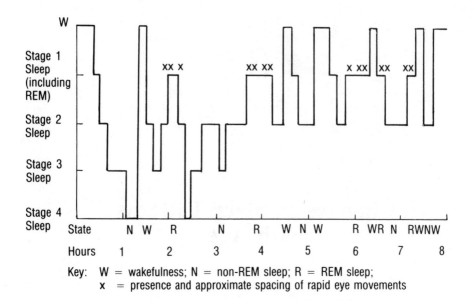

Figure 4. Stages of sleep in a sixty-year-old woman

First of all, let's look at a "hypnogram," or all-night sleep pattern, obtained in a sleep laboratory from a sixty-year-old woman (see figure 4) and compare it with the pattern of the typical young adult we looked at in the last chapter. (Both patterns were obtained in people who had adapted to the sleep laboratory—who had slept there for several nights previously; therefore, they do not represent unusual sleep in persons who are sleeping in a strange place for the first time. We have evidence to indicate that the sleep pattern after several nights in the laboratory is close to the normal pattern a person has at home.)

The differences that stand out are, first of all, that for the sixty-year-old there are several awakenings during the night—five awakenings in this particular case. However, her initial waking period—known as sleep latency, or time to get to sleep—is not especially long, perhaps twenty to thirty minutes. This woman spent a total of just over an hour awake during the night. The next finding that stands out is that this sixty-year-old woman had less deep, slow-wave sleep—stage 4 sleep—than the "typical young adult." Finally, though less prominent, she had somewhat less REM sleep (dreaming sleep), and it is broken up by awakenings.

Everyone is different, but the changes noted in the diagram are some of the most common ones, and all occur quite frequently in the older population. Scientists do not classify these changes as sleep problems, nor do most people who notice them. This sixty-year-old woman, for instance, volunteered to have her sleep studied in the sleep laboratory. She had no particular complaints about her sleep.

TOTAL SLEEP TIME

Now let us look in more detail at some of the important aspects of sleep, or sleep variables, and examine how they change through the human life span. Let us first compare total sleep time in various age groups from birth to age seventy-five (figure 5). This figure and subsequent figures are derived from detailed studies of groups of males and females of different ages sleeping in the laboratory studied by Doctors Robert Williams and Ismet Karacan. These researchers studied at least ten males and ten females at approximately ages four, seven, eleven, fourteen, seventeen, twenty-four, thirty-five, forty-five, fifty-five, sixty-five, and seventy-five. Their conclusions have been confirmed by studies at other laboratories.

The first thing we notice about total sleep time is that it falls dramatically from birth to age twenty. This is something we all know. The newborn spends over twelve hours asleep, and the four-year-olds in the study slept over ten hours. By the age of eighteen or twenty, sleep time is just over seven hours. Average sleep time

Total Sleep Time
(hours)

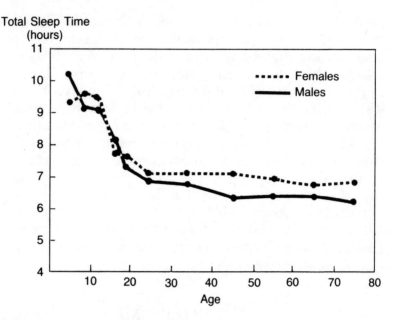

Figure 5. Average hours of sleep, males and females, from birth
to age seventy-five

does not change a tremendous amount from age fifteen
to age seventy-five. On the average, there is a slight
decrease in sleep time.

Although not shown in the figures, the variation
between people increases a great deal with age. For
instance, both the twenty-four-year-old males and the
seventy-five-year-old males slept a little over seven
hours. The average sleep time was only ten minutes
less in the seventy-five-year-olds. However, there was a
great deal of variation among the seventy-five-year-
olds. Whereas the fifteen-year-olds all slept around
seven to eight hours, some of the seventy-five-year-old
men slept five to six hours, and others slept nine to ten
hours, though the average came out to just over seven
hours. Another factor suggests that there may be even
less difference between the age groups: In these studies, subjects were asked not to take naps during the

course of the study. However, it is quite probable that a few brief naps were nonetheless taken by the seventy-five-year-old group. These naps were not included in "total sleep time," since the subjects were recorded only at night. Thus, if we had been able to take those naps into account, the average sleep time might have been almost identical in the older and younger groups.

Finally, the graph shows that there is very little difference in total sleep time between men and women. At ages forty and fifty, women sleep a little more than men on the average, but these differences are not clear-cut either in the younger or older groups.

Total sleep time, therefore, is not something that changes a great deal in older adults. Very definite changes are found, however, in number of awakenings, amount of time awake, and degree of "sleep efficiency," which is the percentage of time in bed actually spent asleep—total sleep time divided by total time in bed.

NUMBER OF AWAKENINGS

Figure 6 shows changes in the number of awakenings in these same groups of people. Just about everyone has one or two brief awakenings during the night. Thus, even the twenty-four-year-old group and the thirty-five-year-old group have an average of one to three awakenings per night. Also, it is clear that the number of awakenings does not change much from childhood through age thirty-five. From age thirty-five on, however, the average number of awakenings during the night increases slightly so that by the age of seventy-five the number of awakenings is about seven per night.

At all ages except age seventy-five, men seem to awaken slightly more on the average than do women, but this is probably not an important difference. It should also be remembered that this graph refers to

Awakenings

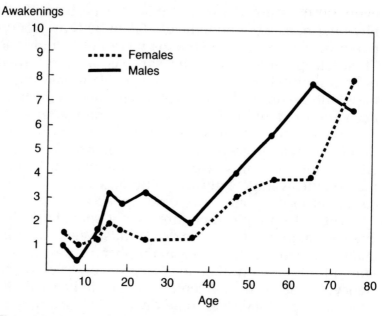

Figure 6. Average number of awakenings during the night, males and females, from birth to age seventy-five

awakenings recorded in the sleep laboratory and may not correspond exactly to awakenings that you remember in the morning. Good sleepers, people who basically do not have sleep complaints, usually underestimate the number of times they awaken. Thus, a typical thirty-five-year-old who awoke twice according to the EEG record may well feel he or she slept all night, and the typical seventy-five-year-old who awoke seven times may feel that he or she awoke only three or four times during the night.

WAKING TIME

Figure 7 shows waking time during the night. This is the percentage of time in bed (excluding time before sleep onset or after final awakening) that is spent awake. Again, only after age forty do these persons without sleep problems show much increase in waking time. People under age forty spend only 1 to 2 percent of their time in bed awake. The amount of waking time begins to increase at age forty and continues to increase, so even a healthy seventy-five-year-old spends 12 to 15 percent of time in bed awake. This is far more

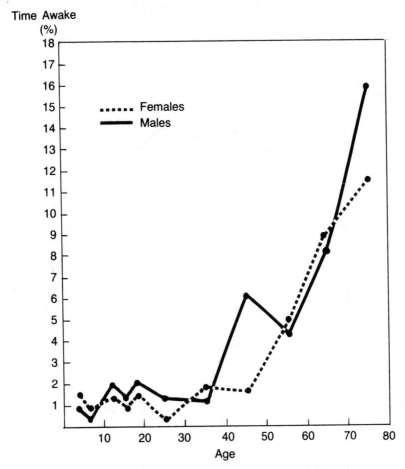

Figure 7. Average time in bed spent awake after initial sleep onset, males and females, from birth to age seventy-five

time than the young adult spends awake, but it nonetheless represents for these subjects slightly less than
one hour of total time in bed.

SLEEP EFFICIENCY

Figure 8 presents "sleep efficiency" (the percentage of
time in bed spent asleep) across the life span. This is
another way of expressing the amount of wakefulness
while in bed. Sleep efficiency falls after age thirty-five

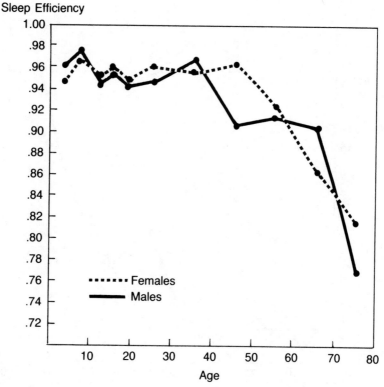

Figure 8. Average proportion of time in bed spent asleep (sleep
efficiency), males and females, from birth to age
seventy-five

and falls approximately equally in men and women. Even in the seventy-five-year-olds, however, approximately 80 percent of the time in bed was spent asleep, and this represented close to six hours of sleep.

SLEEP LATENCY

The time taken to fall asleep, known as sleep latency, reveals an interesting pattern (see figure 9). Again, men and women do not differ particularly. There is actually a slight decrease in the average sleep latency from childhood up to age thirty-five. A thirty-five-year-old falls asleep more quickly, on the average, than does a child or an adolescent. After this, the level remains the same, with sleep latencies of ten to fifteen minutes at ages

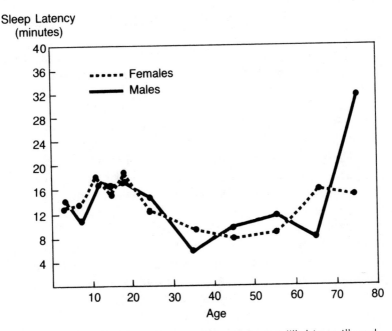

Figure 9. Average sleep latency (time between "lights out" and sleep onset), males and females, from birth to age seventy-five

forty-five, fifty-five, and sixty-five. Only in the oldest group does sleep latency increase, and it seems to do so more in men than in women.

The figures so far have dealt with the basic sleep and wakefulness variables; they have confirmed the impressions obtained from simply asking people about their sleep. As we get older, especially after age forty, we awaken more times and spend more time awake and thus are awake a somewhat greater proportion of the time we are in bed. However, it is worth noting that neither total sleep time nor time taken to fall asleep changes very much. Overall, some changes are clearly present, but data show that there is great variation from person to person. Even among the sixty-five- and the seventy-five-year-olds, there were people whose sleep was hardly different from that of a twenty-five-year-old.

STAGES OF SLEEP

Now, let us examine the sleep data in more detail and look at changes in the stages of sleep, discussed in the last chapter. Figures 10, 11, 12, and 13 can be examined together. What they show is that the amount of time spent in the lighter stages of non-REM sleep, especially stage 1, definitely increases with age. Stage 1 can be considered "dozing" or "just barely sleeping." The amount of time spent in this very light stage of sleep definitely increases with age and increases more in men than in women, consistent with the idea that we get generally "lighter" sleep as we get older. There are fewer definite changes in the amount of stage 2 sleep— only a slight increase with age. The amount of stage 3 and stage 4 sleep, the deepest stages of non-REM sleep, definitely decreases with age. In fact, the change in the very deepest sleep stage, stage 4, is the most dramatic. It falls from about 18 percent of total sleep in the adolescent or young adult to almost none at ages sixty-five and seventy-five. This decrease in stage 3 and stage 4

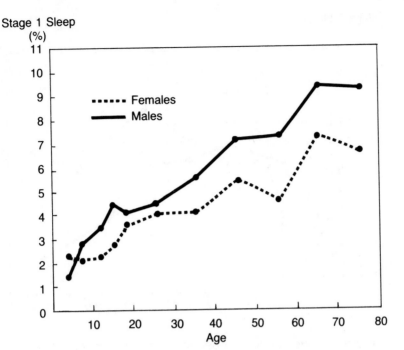

Figure 10. Average time in bed spent in stage 1 sleep, males and females, from birth to age seventy-five

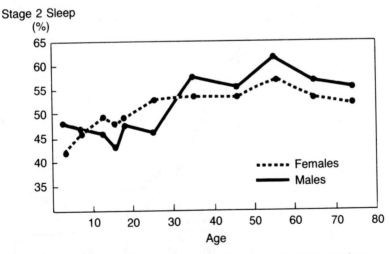

Figure 11. Average time in bed spent in stage 2 sleep, males and females, from birth to age seventy-five

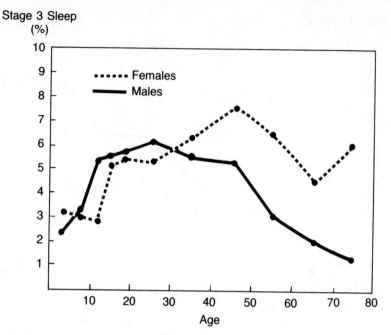

Figure 12. Average time in bed spent in stage 3 sleep, males and females, from birth to age seventy-five

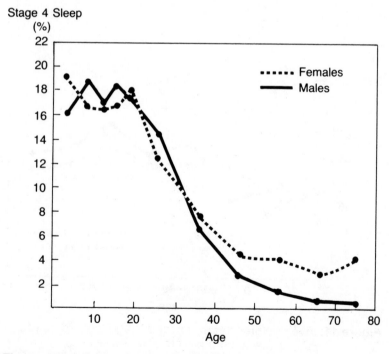

Figure 13. Average time in bed spent in stage 4 sleep, males and females, from birth to age seventy-five

sleep, especially stage 4 sleep, has been noted over and over in many studies and is probably the most clear-cut sleep change occurring with age. It is of interest that the amount of stage 4 sleep drops even more rapidly in men than in women. In terms of sleep—especially the stage 3 and stage 4 changes, but to some extent also the increased light sleep and the changes in wakefulness—men can be said to "age" somewhat more rapidly than women.

Figure 14 represents changes in REM time—time spent in rapid eye movement, or dreaming, sleep. This variable decreases slowly with age, but the chief decrease occurs between birth and age twenty. There is only a very slight decrease from age twenty to age seventy-five.

The facts about changes in sleep stages are clear and well established. Exactly what they mean is not as certain. Possibly the changes are unimportant. Some

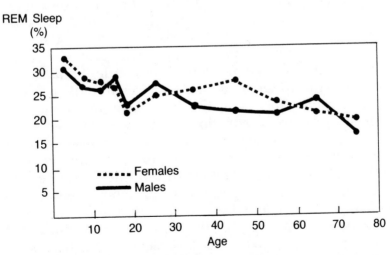

Figure 14. Average time in bed spent in REM sleep, males and females, from birth to age seventy-five

researchers have argued that the change responsible for reduced stage 4 on the recording is simply a slight decrease in the average size of the brain or a slight thickening of the skull resulting in greater distance between the brain itself and the recording electrodes on the scalp. This distance factor in itself can produce a reduction in the number of waves large enough to qualify for stage 4 sleep. However, this is not the entire explanation. Another possibility is that this reduction could be seen simply as secondary to other well-known changes in bodily activity. Many studies of animals and young humans show that stage 4 sleep increases somewhat after bodily activity or exercise (though there is still some disagreement on this point). The reduction of stage 4 sleep with age could be a reflection of the fact that older people are on the average less physically active.

Stage 4 changes may represent something more significant—some sort of measure of aging in the brain. In favor of this is the fact that older people who appear to have aged especially fast have even less stage 3 and stage 4 sleep than other people of the same age.

If we accept that stage 4 reduction may be a measure of aging, or a basic part of aging, a further question concerns cause and effect. Does a reduction of stage 4 sleep simply *reflect* some "aging" changes in the brain? Or does the change in sleep to some extent *cause* other aging changes? Or are both true? It seems quite possible that certain changes in the brain that we cannot yet specify produce a reduction in the synchronized slow-wave activity, which we record as stage 4 sleep. Since we consider stage 4 to be an important restorative part of sleep—associated with growth-hormone release, and probably increased synthesis of proteins—getting less stage 4 sleep could lead to loss of these restorative functions. This suggests the intriguing possibility that attempting to increase stage 4 sleep might help slow down some of the changes of aging. However, this is speculative as yet.

PHYSIOLOGY OF SLEEP

In addition to age-related changes in sleep already discussed, a few specific aspects of the physiology of sleep should be mentioned. Breathing during sleep is a very important dimension of sleep that definitely changes with age. Sleep apnea, a condition in which breathing stops a number of times during the night, can be quite dangerous (see chapter 7). Recent research shows that most of us have occasional "respiratory instability" during sleep and some apneic episodes as we reach our fifties. This condition becomes increasingly common with advancing age.

One recent study demonstrates that by age seventy, over 20 percent of us have significant apnea— more than five apneic episodes per hour. An important question is whether this should be considered simply a normal, inevitable part of the aging process about which one should not worry, or whether it is something that, though common, can be considered pathological and should be treated. This is not a purely theoretical question. A doctor who chooses the second alternative could try to treat the apnea to see whether improved daytime functioning and less daytime tiredness might ensue. Certainly there is evidence that when a person has unusually severe apnea, considerably more than the average, treating the apnea does help daytime functioning. And there is a study indicating that even among older people without severe apnea, those with relatively more respiratory problems at night are sleepier in the daytime. Thus, an older person with severe daytime sleepiness and apnea can be helped by treatment.

It is possible, though not proven, that the large group of older persons with an averge amount of apnea for their age and an average amount of daytime tiredness might also get some help from treatment of the apnea. At the moment, the answer is unclear, but a number of methods are available for treatment of sleep apnea. Anyone who is concerned that this aspect of nighttime sleep is interfering with daytime functioning should consult a physician or a sleep disorders center to get more information, diagnosis, and, if necessary, treatment.

Finally, there is one aspect of sleep in males that does not change a great deal with age. Penile erections are a regular part of REM sleep, and most adult males have three or four full or partial erections during every night. There is good evidence that this pattern does not change a great deal with age. Dr. Charles Fisher and his colleagues at Mount Sinai Hospital in New York City have obtained data on a number of men in their nineties demonstrating fairly normal patterns of erection.

In this chapter, we have examined how sleep and a number of aspects of sleep change as the human being ages. It appears that much changes, but much also remains the same. Being awake more times during the night than you used to be, spending more time lying in bed not sleeping, and experiencing lighter sleep are changes expected with age and need not be a source of worry.

I asked a very cheerful eighty-five-year-old woman I know about changes in her sleep, thinking that since she seemed so well and active, perhaps she was an exception—someone whose sleep had not changed with age. However, this was not the case. She smiled and said, "When I stop to think about it, my sleep isn't quite the way it was, but neither is my sight, my hearing, my appetite, or anything else. We are not expected to stay exactly the same forever, are we?"

◀ 4 ▶

Diagnosing Sleep Disorders—Self-Help or Professional Help

Since sleep occupies one-third of our lives and consists of two states, the possibilities for disorders of sleep to arise are many. One finding from a number of recent studies is that the control of the body's physiological functions is totally different during sleep than during wakefulness and sometimes differs even between the two major sleep states, non-REM sleep and REM sleep. Those differences provide an opportunity for many specific disorders of the sleep mechanisms to appear and also result in the possibility of secondary disorders; for example, various chemical and environmental stimuli may have different effects during sleep than they do during wakefulness and may, thus, unexpectedly produce sleep disorders.

The field of sleep disorders, or sleep disorders medicine, therefore, is at present rapidly expanding. Masses of data are accumulating about an increasing number of conditions, and there is some disagreement

39

as to how the many clinical conditions related to sleep can be organized and classified. (See Appendix A for an adapted outline of the diagnostic classifications developed by the Association of Sleep Disorders Centers.) There are only a few sleep symptoms but many causes for each symptom. A symptom is a complaint—"I can't fall asleep," "My head aches," and so on. One should not confuse a symptom with an underlying disease. For example, one should not assume that insomnia, trouble sleeping, is a disease that should be "cured" by taking a sleeping pill. Rather, insomnia is a symptom that can be caused by many different diseases and underlying conditions.

Before approaching the question of whether you have a particular sleep disorder, you have to decide whether your sleep problem is serious enough to warrant investigation. Is waking three times a night serious? Is snoring serious? Is sleeping only five hours out of twenty-four serious? We all awake occasionally during the night, and we all awake more during the night as we get older. This is not in itself something to worry about. But beyond this, how does one decide whether the problem is serious? The question is not easy to answer, and there is considerable disagreement between professionals. Overall, no absolute standards can be applied. In terms of length of sleep, for example, there are persons who always sleep four to six hours a night and can function well. They are not insomniacs; they have no particular complaints; they simply require less sleep than most of us.

How then do you decide whether your sleep problem is serious? The important issue is not so much what happens at night but what happens during the day. For example, you always slept well, had no problems, and felt fine during the day until six months ago. Now you are sleeping less and less at night, you are awake more and more, you are so tired in the daytime that you cannot do your work, you are about to get fired, and you fell asleep at the wheel last week and had a bad accident. This adds up to a serious problem with which you need help.

In other words, you need help if your sleep disorder appears to be producing problems with your life—problems in working, interacting with other people, and feeling good in the daytime. (Also, you need help if your sleep disorder produces difficulty in heart or lung functioning or increased blood pressure.) If you simply can't seem to get over six hours of sleep or you awake four times every night, there is not necessarily anything to worry about. It depends on how you function in the daytime.

People differ considerably in their tendency to seek help. Some people are "overworriers"; even minor complaints are cause for running to see a doctor. Other people are "underworriers"; they can be very sick indeed without ever seeking help. It is important to look at your overall health and your daytime functioning. Ask others around you how they evaluate your functioning. If you are enjoying life, enjoying the people around you, and working well or functioning well at whatever you do in the daytime (in Freud's phrase, health involves the ability to "work well and love well"), and if your last physical exam indicated that your body was in good shape, your sleep problem is not a major concern.

SLEEP HYGIENE

If you decide that you do *not* have a really serious sleep problem that requires medical consultation, this doesn't mean that you cannot do anything for yourself. If you have insomnia, the most common symptom, you may want to try one or more of the following sleep hygiene measures on a trial-and-error basis; one of them could solve your problem, and they won't hurt, except insofar

SLEEP HYGIENE

One or more of the following suggestions may be helpful to you.

Do—

• go to bed at a regular time each night.

• get up at approximately the same time each morning.

• eat meals at regular times.

• exercise at regular times (moderate, regular exercise two to four hours before bedtime is especially helpful).

• sleep in a darkened room.

• eliminate noise in the sleeping area.

• eliminate lumps in the bed.

• use a mattress that is neither too soft nor too hard.

• avoid using uncomfortable pillows.

• be sure the room is free of known allergens.

• adjust the temperature to be the most comfortable for you.

• get out of bed if you can't fall asleep after a reasonable amount of time.

• read, listen to music, or watch TV (but not in bed) if you can't fall asleep.

• drink a glass of warm milk or have a light snack before going to bed if you have found this useful in the past.

Don't—

• change your sleep schedule from day to day if you can help it.

• take sleeping pills or other medications that have not been specifically prescribed for you.

• eat a large meal just before bedtime.

• exercise just before you go to bed.

• drink any caffeinated beverages after noon.

• use alcohol to help you sleep.

• go to bed if you are not tired.

• eat or drink in bed.

• read in bed.

• watch TV in bed.

• argue with bedmate or others in bed.

• stay in bed if you can't fall asleep.

as they could delay professional treatment if you should need it.

Regular Bedtimes and Waking Times

It is generally a good idea to adopt a regular sleeping and waking schedule. This almost always helps your body sleep. Sometimes it is all you need. Generally, increasing your time in bed is not helpful in improving sleep. In most cases, if you try to give yourself more time in bed so that you will get more sleep, what you will accomplish is simply spending more time awake in bed feeling uncomfortable and restless. You will gradually associate your bed with a place where you feel uncomfortable, and your mild sleep problem will not improve and may even become worse. So go to bed at the same time every night and don't spend too much time in bed—seven or seven-and-one-half hours is usually enough. And although I do not usually recommend daytime sleep, some older people may find they feel refreshed and function better with a twenty- to sixty-minute nap in the middle of the day. There is nothing wrong with this. However, if such is the case with you, remember that your body will perform better if you schedule this nap at a regular time and do not simply take a nap whenever you feel tired.

Restricted Use of Your Bed

Unless you are very ill and need to spend your time in bed, consider your bed a place to sleep only—and maybe a place for making love. If you have insomnia, don't spend a lot of time eating in bed, watching TV in bed, or lying in bed worrying. Eat, watch TV, and worry somewhere else. This will help your body associate your bed with sleep rather than with waking activities.

Regular Mealtimes

Keep your mealtimes regular. Avoid large meals at bedtime. Here again, people differ considerably; but, for most people, a large and difficult-to-digest meal at bedtime makes sleeping more difficult. Also, sugars and some other carbohydrates taken at bedtime may occasionally produce uncomfortable awakenings an hour or two later, accompanied by the feeling that "something is wrong." On the other hand, this does not mean that you must eat absolutely nothing close to bedtime. You have to find what's right for you. Some people do best eating nothing whatever after dinner; others do well with a small snack at bedtime or close to bedtime.

Exercise

Do a little exercise in the early evening or late afternoon if possible. Exercise in itself can be a useful remedy for insomnia, especially for difficulty in falling asleep. The most helpful form is regular mild-to-moderate exercise done two to four hours before sleep (not just before going to bed and not just after a meal). The kind of exercise doesn't matter much; choose something you'll be comfortable doing every day, not something that feels like torture.

Quiet and Comfortable Bedroom

Make your bedroom as quiet and peaceful as possible. Some people—and you may be one of them—are especially sensitive to various sleep-disturbing factors such as light, noise, lumps in the bed, beds that are too hard or too soft, uncomfortable pillows, and allergens. If you are one of these people, it is certainly worth changing the environment—sealing windows, wearing black patches over your eyes, using a gadget that makes "white noise" to drown out other noises, and so on. Get a bed and a pillow that seem most comfortable to you and also adjust your room temperature so that you feel comfortable; some people sleep best when the temperature is over 70° F. Some people require gadgets or changes to improve their sleep. It's your body and it's your sleep. If something works, do it!

SYMPTOMS, SIGNS, AND CAUSES

If you should decide that you *do* have a serious problem, whether your complaint is insomnia, excessive daytime sleepiness, or something else, the next step is a careful diagnosis, which means an attempt to find out what factors are responsible for the complaint. To a certain extent, you can do this yourself; in many cases, however, you will need the help of your physician and sometimes of a sleep disorders specialist or a psychiatrist. Keeping a sleep log for at least two weeks can yield information that can be helpful for both you and, if necessary, your physician (see pages 46–47).

In attempting to make a diagnosis, you will need to distinguish between symptom, sign, and cause. A symptom is just a complaint: "I can't get to sleep at night"; "I feel hot and flushed"; "My back aches." A sign is a "complaint" that is not made by the patient but by someone nearby or by an instrument: "He doesn't know it, but he falls asleep all the time"; "He snores heavily at night"; "She has a temperature of between 101 and 102° F every afternoon." The important point is that one should not treat a symptom or a sign as though it were a disease (an underlying cause) and immediately go ahead and "cure" it.

If you have a serious fever, a good doctor will try to find out what is causing the fever rather than simply give you an aspirin to reduce it. There are hundreds of possible causes. The fever may be caused by pneumococcal pneumonia, in which case a specific antibiotic is the proper treatment. It may be caused by malaria, which requires other medication. Or your fever may be caused by a respiratory virus, in which case no specific treatment is needed; you can simply wait a week or two for it to go away (and meanwhile aspirin will be useful in making you feel better). The situation is similar with sleep problems. When someone says to me, "I can't sleep," I do not simply say, "Take a sleeping pill." This would be treating the symptom without knowing the

SLEEP LOG

Date	Time You Went to Bed	Time You Got Up	Amount of Time Taken to Fall Asleep	Number of Awakenings During the Night

Time Taken to Fall Asleep Again (Average)	Number of Hours Slept	How You Feel the Following Day 0–5 (0 = Not Rested At All 5 = Well Rested)	Time Slept During the Day (When and How Long)	All Medications Taken

cause. When we look for the cause, we usually find a disease or a condition, which then has its own treatment. In the next chapters, we will consider the chief causes of insomnia and other symptoms.

THE SLEEP DISORDERS CENTER

When a sleeping problem appears to be potentially serious, your physician may ask you to see a sleep disorders specialist at a sleep disorders center.

Most sleep disorders centers are quite small, so you will receive considerable personal attention. The specialist generally spends forty to sixty minutes getting a detailed description and history of your problem. The doctor asks questions about any medical illnesses and about any periods of mental disturbance, depression, or anxiety. He or she asks about your medications and habits, such as smoking or drinking. The doctor may ask something about your family, your waking life— whether you are tired in the daytime, have any unusual episodes of sleepiness in the daytime, and so on.

Then, depending on what is found in this initial interview, the specialist may recommend further tests and studies. Sometimes the doctor will be able to make suggestions to help you immediately after this first visit. More frequently, the doctor will ask you to fill out some medical and psychological questionnaires and may ask you to come to the sleep center for an all-night sleep recording—a polysomnographic study—or for some daytime sleep studies.

An all-night sleep study does not usually involve a hospital admission. It simply involves going to a sleep center an hour or two before your normal sleep time. There, you are "hooked up" for the study. This involves a lot of wires, but nothing painful. Information is transmitted through the wires *from* you, the sleeper, *to* a recording machine. Nothing goes *to* the body. You do not receive shocks or painful sensations of any kind. No needles are used. What happens is simply that small discs, electrodes, are pasted on your head, the side of your face, and usually your chest and legs as well. These electrodes allow the technician to record from the surface of your skin evidence of brain waves, eye movements, and muscle potential. Usually respiration and pulse rate are also recorded throughout the night. Often, you will be asked to wear a light mask to help in the recording of respiration and breathing and sometimes a clip on your finger or your ear that will help in measuring oxygen saturation. The technician is present all night long in a room next to you to monitor the recordings.

A few centers make it possible for you to have home monitoring—sleep recording done in your own home. However, the technology for home monitoring is still being developed, and, at the moment, it is beset by

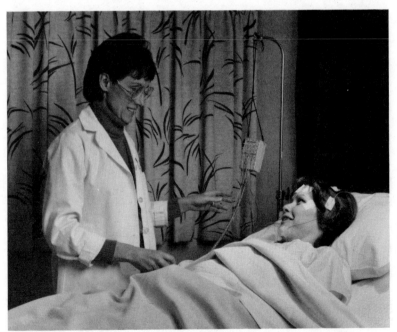

Preparing a patient for a sleep study at the Newton-Wellesley Hospital Sleep Disorders Center

a number of problems. Although home monitoring sounds simpler and more comfortable than being monitored at a sleep center, many wires and sensing devices must be attached to you in both settings. If the record is not made at a center, someone from the center has to come and attach the wires at your home; you cannot do it yourself. Your recording is then made on tape at your bedside or transmitted by telephone wires to the laboratory. If some minor difficulty arises during the night, there is no one there who can make a simple adjustment. Thus, a minor problem that could easily be fixed in the laboratory may make the home recording impossible to read, and it will have to be repeated.

The specialist spends a good deal of time looking over the nighttime sleep recording as well as any other tests that may be taken, such as a daytime recording or, when indicated, certain psychological tests. Usually by

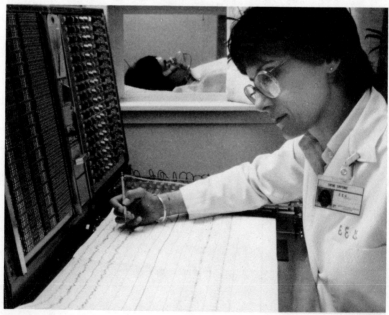

A sleep recording at the Newton-Wellesley Hospital Sleep Disorders Center

the second or third meeting with you, the doctor can determine what is wrong and what can be done about it.

The sleep disorders specialist will probably make a diagnosis of your sleep problem using the classification developed by the Association for Sleep Disorders Centers. (See Appendix A for a simplified version of this classification.) Should you ever decide to visit a sleep disorders center, you may want to look over this classification yourself; you may get some ideas of where your problem fits into the outline, and looking at it may provide you with some questions to ask the specialist. (The conditions in this outline that affect older persons will be discussed in the next five chapters.)

Treatment sometimes involves changes in daytime activities. It can involve taking a new medication or stopping an old one. Sometimes it will involve suggestions for psychotherapy or other forms of psychological intervention. Sometimes there is need for further medical consultation and even for surgery. The specialist will discuss these alternatives in detail with you and perhaps with a family member as well.

Most people have found that spending the night at a sleep disorders center is not painful or unpleasant, though it is certainly a new and different experience, and occasionally a person may find the wires and equipment a bit frightening. The accommodations are usually comfortable, and there is someone with you all night (in the next room) should you need anything. The cost is generally covered by insurance. If your doctor does not know of a sleep disorders center near you, show him or her the listing in Appendix B. Sleep disorders specialists are listed in Appendix C.

◀ 5 ▶

Insomnia:
Medical Causes

Of the symptoms associated with sleep disorders, by far the most common is insomnia. Insomnia is manifested by any one or more of a group of related complaints: "I have trouble falling asleep. I stay awake for hours." "I have trouble remaining asleep. I keep waking up during the night." "I wake up and I just can't get back to sleep." "I wake up much earlier than I want to." All of these together constitute insomnia.

Basically, one can think of insomnia as consisting of two different and usually separable symptoms: difficulty in falling asleep and difficulty in remaining asleep. Difficulty in falling asleep is very common in young people but is found in older persons as well.

Difficulty in remaining asleep, which can consist of awaking frequently during the night or awaking too early in the morning, is an even more common symptom in older people than is difficulty in falling asleep. Insomnia can result from a variety of medical and psychological causes as well and from insufficient daytime activity and poor sleep hygiene.

PAINFUL CONDITIONS

One of the most common medical causes of insomnia in older persons is pain. If you have arthritis, for example, it can flare up repeatedly, producing a painful sensation in one or more joints, despite a variety of useful treatments. When you roll over during the night, the affected joint registers pain, and the pain wakes you up. Of course pain and discomfort can also make it hard to fall asleep in the first place. People who are active or busy in the daytime will sometimes ignore a minor ache, which then suddenly becomes unbearable in the evening when they are lying in bed with nothing to distract them. Obviously, if the pain is causing you insomnia, the best approach is to determine what is causing the pain and obtain treatment for that condition.

SLEEP APNEA

One very important but often unrecognized medical cause of insomnia is sleep apnea, in which sleep is disturbed repeatedly because the breathing apparatus is not working well. This cause is often not at all apparent to the sleeper, the person who has the problem. He or she may simply say, "I fall asleep all right, but I wake up a lot, and I'm tired in the daytime." However, someone else watching the sleeper—a spouse, bedmate, or roommate—will say, "He sleeps terribly; he snores heavily and then stops snoring; he gasps, chokes, at times seems not to be breathing at all," and so on. To be certain about this condition, one needs to see a sleep specialist and have one or more all-night sleep recordings made. (Sleep apnea can be a very serious condition; since it produces a complaint of daytime sleepiness more often than a complaint of insomnia, it will be discussed in more detail in chapter 7.)

MYOCLONUS

Another serious and sometimes related medical condition is known as nocturnal myoclonus, or periodic movements during sleep. The person suffering from it may report waking up frequently every night or may not notice anything much except waking up tired in the morning or being tired in the daytime—in other words, having "nonrestorative sleep." Occasionally, she—this condition is somewhat more common in women than in men—may notice that her arms or legs move around or make jerking movements. Often, she will report strange bits of dreams on awaking—sometimes very active bits: "I was jumping over a stream . . . something like that . . . and I woke up." "Something suddenly came into the room. I leaped back and woke up."

Most of us occasionally have such experiences as we are falling asleep. But if they happen a lot and seem to interfere with sleep, something is not right. In trying to diagnose this condition, getting information from the bedmate or roommate is extremely useful. The other person, assuming he or she does not sleep too deeply, will say something like this: "Yes, you know she seems to be asleep, but for long periods her legs have these jerky movements. Sometimes her whole body jerks. She half wakes up and then goes back to sleep again. Sometimes this happens for hours. It's amazing she can get any sleep." If this individual is recorded in the sleep laboratory, one sees a very clear-cut pattern of myoclonic jerks—muscle jerks occurring every thirty to sixty seconds for hours, sometimes throughout the night.

Although nocturnal myoclonus is one of the underlying causes of insomnia and of daytime sleepiness, one can go further and try to find an underlying cause for the myoclonus. Sometimes it accompanies other conditions, such as sleep apnea. It can be produced by chemical imbalances, such as occur with severe liver or kidney disease; and it can occasionally be a side effect of various medications. But in many cases we simply consider it a neuromuscular hypersensitivity or hyperactivity, since we cannot determine any other cause.

To make certain that nocturnal myoclonus exists and to determine its severity, all-night sleep recordings are needed. The sleep disorders specialist must remember that the simple presence of myoclonus is not necessarily cause for concern. It is when myoclonus produces awakenings, poor sleep, and excessive daytime sleepiness that it should be treated. Many older persons have some jerking movements of the legs during sleep that do not necessarily produce any noticeable insomnia or daytime sleepiness. However, excessive daytime sleepiness can sometimes be clearly related to hundreds of jerking movements during the night, which make it impossible for the person to obtain periods of continuous sleep, even though she or he spends eight or more hours in bed every night. Treatment of the myoclonus, using medication, can allow the patient to sleep well again and, thus, clear up the daytime sleepiness.

Treatment of myoclonus will depend on whether the myoclonus is secondary to another condition. When one of these conditions is present, it should be treated or changed first. When one of these is not present or cannot be treated, the myoclonus can be treated independently by one of several medications.

People who have myoclonus at night often have a daytime condition called restless legs syndrome. This is just what it sounds like—your muscles feel uncomfortable and restless. You do not have real pain, but when you sit or lie down for a prolonged period, you feel you have to move your legs. Restless legs syndrome is probably caused by the same neuromuscular sensitivity that causes the muscle jerks at night. Anyone with serious restless legs syndrome in the daytime should be checked to determine whether nocturnal myoclonus is also present.

MENOPAUSAL CHANGES

Insomnia related to menopause, or perimenopausal insomnia, is not listed officially as a sleep disorder, but it is a common condition that deserves to be recognized and studied further. In women around age fifty, there are often complaints of insomnia as part of a more general syndrome of bodily changes around or shortly after menopause. The hormonal changes of this period are sometimes associated with the well-known hot flashes and sometimes with sweating, muscle aches, anxiety, and agitation. When these symptoms occur at night, they can seriously disturb sleep. This is one aspect of the insomnia, but there can be more to it than that. At the time of menopause, some women suffer serious insomnia probably related to changes in brain biochemistry involving serotonin and other substances that can directly affect sleep.

Perimenopausal insomnia is usually not severe, and a woman is usually able to fall asleep again after the disruption. If the insomnia becomes increasingly severe, with serious early morning wakefulness or many awakenings during the night, tiredness in the daytime, and being unable to function in the morning, other causes of the insomnia—especially depression—must be considered.

In terms of treatment, the woman, together with her physician, can decide whether the overall symptoms are serious enough to warrant use of estrogen replacement therapy. Often estrogen will reduce all the symptoms of menopause, including the insomnia; however, there are risks in taking estrogen that must be carefully considered.

A group in England has been experimenting with the amino acid tryptophan to treat groups of women suffering from depression and insomnia around the time of menopause. The use of tryptophan with this particular group of problems is not yet well established. But this food substance can help one fall asleep faster and reduce wakefulness. One or two grams (1,000 or 2,000 milligrams) taken forty-five minutes before bedtime should be adequate.

In the United States, tryptophan can be purchased as a food substance at vitamin and health food stores, but it cannot at the moment be prescribed as a drug. In Europe, where it is actually prescribed for sleep, doctors usually recommend taking it three or four nights a week and then not taking it for the remainder of the week; they find it works even better this way than it does when taken every night. However, don't take anything, even tryptophan, for long periods without consulting your physician.

MEDICATION AND DRUGS

Another frequent and little-recognized cause of insomnia is prescribed medication. It is unfortunate but true that hardly any of the wonderful drugs discovered by modern medicine are free of side effects and problems. There is almost always a price to pay, and sleep problems are in many cases part of the price. This is a complex issue, since there are hundreds of drugs involved, but there are a few general principles.

First, there are drugs that actually have a stimulant effect and that will produce difficulty in sleeping as a direct pharmacologic effect, especially if taken in the evening. These include the amphetamines (Dexedrine, Eskatrol), methylphenidate (Ritalin), pemoline (Cylert), and many similar drugs used to treat narcolepsy and other medical conditions and, occasionally, obesity. Cocaine is a stimulant, too, quite similar to the amphetamines.

These are the well-recognized stimulants; however, there are many groups of drugs that only have stimulant effects under certain conditions or only have them in certain sensitive people. These include monoamine oxidase inhibitors such as phenelzine (Nardil) and tranylcypromine (Parnate), sometimes used as antidepressants, and levodopa (Larodopa, Dopar) and related drugs used to treat Parkinsonism. If a stimulant drug is responsible for insomnia, the problem can sometimes be improved by reducing the dose of medicine, by taking the medication earlier in the day, or by changing to another medication.

Caffeine, one of the world's most widely used mild stimulants, can also interfere with sleep. Most of us drink some coffee or tea without considering that we are taking a drug, since it is just part of the meal. However, our brains and bodies do not make this distinction. Caffeine, if taken in large enough doses, has effects on the brain very similar to those produced by stimulants such as amphetamines or cocaine.

Most of us get along perfectly well ingesting small amounts of caffeine every day, but several points are worth keeping in mind. First of all, we should be aware that caffeine is contained not only in coffee but in tea, cola drinks, and hot chocolate. It is harder to calculate the amount in a cup of tea because people make their tea very differently, but a weak cup of tea will have perhaps half the caffeine of a cup of coffee, while a really strong cup of tea may have almost as much as a cup of coffee.

Secondly, we differ tremendously in our sensitivity to caffeine and, for that matter, in our sensitivity to alcohol and other drugs. So you have to get to know yourself. Some people can drink three, four, five, or more cups of coffee a day—even drink coffee in the evening—and sleep quite well. Others have great trouble falling asleep if they have so much as a single cup of coffee anytime after lunch. And some people who can tolerate a lot of caffeine when young become more sensitive to it as they grow older. If you do have trouble sleeping, especially trouble falling asleep, look at your caffeine consumption; if you think caffeine might be affecting your sleep, it's easy enough to stop for a while and see whether this makes a difference. Cut down on caffeine over a few days; do not stop all at once. Then stay off it for a month or so before you decide whether that has helped.

Surprisingly, the drugs known as sleeping pills or tranquilizers can also produce insomnia! Here, the problem is that there is almost always a rebound—an effect in the opposite direction—when one withdraws from or stops taking the medication. Thus, someone taking a sleeping pill or a tranquilizer for a few weeks to get over a difficult period will then often find some difficulty sleeping when he or she stops. Unfortunately, this pattern is true not only of the older, "heavy" sleeping pills and sedatives such as the barbiturates but also of the benzodiazepines—the most widely used hypnotics and tranquilizers at present, including such prescription medications as diazepam (Valium), chlordiazepoxide (Librium), triazolam (Halcion), temazepam (Restoril), and flurazepam (Dalmane). A period of at least mild and sometimes severe insomnia after withdrawal is expectable, though again people's reactions vary. Some people may scarcely notice it, while some may complain of sleep problems for weeks. The patient, with the help of the physician, needs to find some way to get through this period. The body will readjust in time, though this may sometimes take weeks.

If you are taking medication, either prescription or nonprescription, you will benefit from keeping a chart like the one on pages 62–63. This allows you to record the date you started using each medication, the dosage and schedule, any change in dosage and schedule, and the date you stopped taking the medication. On the same chart you can indicate under Results or Side Effects any sleep-related problems (insomnia, excessive sleepiness, nightmares, etc.) and the dates these symptoms occurred. There is also space for you to record any other disturbing symptoms and the dates they occurred. When you start taking a new medication, enter in the chart the name of the medication, the name of the physician who prescribed it, the place where you purchased it, the prescription number, and the condition for which it was prescribed. Such a chart will be of great help for you and also for your physician in trying to determine whether sleep problems or other problems you are having may be related to medication you are taking.

ALCOHOL

A very frequent cause of insomnia, seldom recognized as such, is alcohol. This may be a surprise to some readers, since alcohol is often used as a sleeping pill. People are told that a little beer or a slug of whiskey at bedtime will help put them to sleep. Alcohol, however, is a great paradox. It is often used as a sleeping pill, and it does have some sleep-inducing effect. Yet alcohol can produce quite serious insomnia and, in fact, two different patterns of insomnia. One can find this out simply by talking in detail with heavy drinkers or alcoholics; one can establish it with certainty in the sleep laboratory. The first pattern often found is that a heavy drinker, whether considered alcoholic or not, will indeed fall asleep quickly but will then awake after four or five hours and often be unable to get back to sleep. As heavy drinking continues, the four- to five-hour sleep period diminishes until finally the drinker is obtaining hardly more than an hour of sleep before the awakenings begin. In addition, the awakenings are sometimes quite unpleasant, associated with frightening feelings and strange bodily sensations.

Name: _____

Medications   Medicines Prescribed by Doctor

Name of Physician, Name of Medication, Place Purchased, and Prescription Number	Reason for Taking Medication	Date Started Taking Medication

Medications   Taken Without Prescription

Name of Medication	Reason for Taking Medication	Date Started Taking Medication

Dosage and Schedule	Any Change in Dosage and Schedule (Include Dates)	Results or Side Effects (Include Dates)	Date Stopped Taking Medication

Dosage and Schedule	Any Change in Dosage and Schedule (Include Dates)	Results or Side Effects (Include Dates)	Date Stopped Taking Medication

Unfortunately, this pattern is not the whole story. When the heavy drinker finally decides to stop drinking, another pattern of insomnia shows up. This is the insomnia found after discontinuation of any depressant or sleeping medication. For at least a week, and sometimes much longer, after one stops drinking, one experiences poor sleep, a feeling of hardly having been asleep, and sleep with a great many dreams and sometimes nightmares continuing throughout the night. It is very important to remember that this is part of withdrawal and will pass after a while.

If you drink intermittently—that is, drink heavily for a week or two and then stop for a while, repeating the sequence—the two patterns of insomnia may become mixed, and after a while you won't know what's going on, but you will know that your sleep has become poor and disturbed. This is one cause of insomnia that you can definitely treat yourself—sometimes with help from friends, from a counselor, and from Alcoholics Anonymous. A sleep specialist won't be of much use, except perhaps in confirming for you that alcohol is the main problem and that you don't have one of the other sleep disorders.

Often alcohol interacts with other causes of insomnia. What happens is something like this:

Joe's wife, Alice, died a year ago. Joe is retired, but he and his wife took part in many activities and had a great many friends. He was living an active, interesting life with his wife. After her death, Joe obtained a good deal of support from their mutual friends and from members of the family, who all took great interest in him. However, over the past year, this interest has gradually diminished. Joe has found that many of the friends he thought were mutual friends were more Alice's friends, and they have now gradually drifted away. Also, the activities he and Alice used to do together, such as attending the theater and visiting museums aren't much fun to do alone.

Joe finds himself with less and less to do. He is already suffering to some extent from insufficient activity, or low-arousal syndrome. He's not very active, involved, or energetic in the daytime and therefore does not sleep as well at night as he used to. In addition, he misses his wife. He has some unresolved grief, perhaps a mild depression. Joe is not someone who talks easily with friends, and he has not obtained the help of a psychotherapist, so his depression stays with him, unresolved. This in turn can negatively affect his sleep, making it more difficult for him to get involved in new activities that might help him. So Joe spends more time alone, relatively inactive and slightly depressed. What does he do with himself? Well, he watches TV a lot. He tries to take walks. He stops in at the local bar and drinks with a few friends and acquaintances he remembers from the old days.

Since there is not much else to do, he increases his visits to his local bar in the evening and drinks more than he used to. He finds that he is not falling asleep as readily as he once did, and he figures an extra shot or two of whiskey will help him fall asleep. Of course, to some extent it does. So although Joe has not had a drinking problem in the past, he is now regularly consuming four, six, or eight drinks per day. This is probably too much alcohol for anyone, but especially for an older person, whose body has become somewhat less able to chemically handle the alcohol or "clear" it from the body.

Joe's problem now is no longer a problem of falling asleep, since the two or three drinks he takes at bedtime are sufficient to knock him out. However, as he continues to drink, he finds he awakes earlier and earlier in the morning; he awakes during the night as well and is unable to get back to sleep. He sleeps restlessly and has had a few episodes in which he woke up screaming or thrashing around in bed. Finally, his friends are concerned enough about his general state of health that they encourage him to seek help.

OTHER MEDICAL CAUSES

The conditions discussed above are the most common medical causes of insomnia in older persons. However, numerous medical illnesses can sometimes be responsible for serious insomnia; for example, hyperthyroidism (overactivity of the thyroid gland) and the opposite condition, hypothyroidism (underactivity of the thyroid gland), can both produce insomnia. The existence of such conditions reinforces the fact that a visit to a physician and a physical examination should be part of your evaluation for serious insomnia.

◀ 6 ▶

Insomnia:
Psychological Causes

In addition to these known and suspected medical causes of insomnia, there are a number of causes of insomnia that can most easily be described using psychological terms, though the body's physiology is definitely involved.

INSUFFICIENT PHYSICAL OR MENTAL ACTIVITY

A very common cause for insomnia in older persons, especially in the years just after retirement or after reducing one's activities for some other reason, is insufficient physical or mental activity. People often find that they don't have much to do after retirement and may spend their days watching TV, sometimes dozing a bit in front of the TV set, and then find that they have trouble falling asleep in the evening. (An example is Daniel, whose sleeping problem was discussed in the first chapter.)

The easiest way to explain this sort of insomnia is simply that it's hard to fall asleep when you're not tired. (It's almost like trying to fall asleep when you've just had a night's sleep.) The solution is straightforward. You have to be active in some way in the daytime in order to become tired out and fall asleep quickly at night. What to do depends on the individual, but in my experience a combination of moderate physical activity—just walking is all right—with some satisfying mental activity works best. Purely mental effort makes you tired, but it can be an irritable tiredness, as in children who become fussy and "too tired to fall asleep."

We all need to do something active with our bodies and our minds. We are more likely to feel a desirable sort of tiredness at the end of the day if we have had some moderate physical activity, some mental activity, and also some emotional satisfaction at having accomplished something during the course of the day. This may sound like a lot to ask of a day, but it need not be. It doesn't mean scheduling a whole series of separate activities. For instance, in some older persons, the simple task of baby-sitting with grandchildren or great-grandchildren (your own or a friend's) may fulfill all these requirements. It often involves quite a bit of physical activity, some mental work—of reading to the children, playing games with them, teaching them things—and certainly the emotional satisfaction of having accomplished something.

ANXIETY

There are many well-recognized psychological causes of insomnia. For instance, different kinds of anxiety clearly produce difficulty in falling asleep. Worry over an upcoming event—a job interview or a move of some kind, for example—can often make it difficult to *fall* asleep rather than to remain asleep. You spend your time thinking—either being excited or worried about what is going to happen. This kind of thing still happens, of course, as one gets older, but it is a more frequent cause of sleeping difficulty in young persons. Older persons who awake a few times each night for other reasons may experience difficulty in falling asleep again after their awakenings when they have this kind of anxiety.

A fairly common cause of insomnia occurring in older persons as well as in younger ones involves a type of anxiety that can be called fear of letting go. A woman who did not seem to have any of the medical causes for insomnia reported that over many years she had had trouble falling asleep and that she would usually become more scared or agitated when she went to bed. It appeared that the process of gradually falling asleep and relaxing was not pleasant for her but was, in fact, very disturbing. Relaxing and going to sleep brought up old, half-forgotten memories of disturbing fights between her parents, a threatening figure of an uncle who may have abused her when she was a child, and a fear that something awful would happen to her at some point while she wasn't looking—while she had "let down her guard." This woman, not surprisingly, also found it hard to relax in social situations, to let down her guard with friends or at a party. What this woman was experiencing involved a fear of letting go. And, of course, since falling asleep is letting go, someone who has such fears will have difficulty falling asleep. This kind of insomnia can often be helped by psychotherapy.

There is another kind of anxiety, more severe, called prepsychotic anxiety, where the increasing anxiety and associated insomnia are early signs of an impending psychosis. This type of anxiety often occurs in a young person—a student, say, who cannot sleep, is

becoming more and more anxious, stops eating, becomes increasingly scared, and has vague terrors and
paranoid feelings. The person finally shows up at a
hospital emergency room acting "crazy"—disorganized
and out of control. Although this happens more frequently in young people, it can definitely occur in older
persons as well, especially those who have a history of
similar episodes. If you or a loved one have an insomnia
associated with anxiety that has come on acutely and is
getting worse over a period of weeks, it is important
that you consult your physician as soon as possible.

Anxiety also plays a part in the causes of the kinds
of insomnia discussed below.

STRESS REACTIONS

Stressful situations of any kind will disrupt the normal
balance of your life, and this disruption can often include insomnia. With luck the reaction will last only a
few days; sometimes it will last for weeks and occasionally months, depending on the nature of the stress and
on the person involved. This condition is known as
transient psychophysiological insomnia. The sleep disturbance produced can be either difficulty falling asleep
or frequent waking during the night and inability to get
back to sleep. In younger persons, it is almost always
the former; in older persons, the difficulty in remaining
asleep may predominate, or both conditions may be
present.

It is worth keeping in mind, of course, that stress is
not an absolute term. What is not stressful for one
person may be very stressful for another; people vary a
good deal in their reactions to stress and change. An
individual's reactions to stress will also vary at different
times in his or her life. For example, when we are thirty,
forty, or fifty, a move from one residence to another
may represent a new job, new challenges, and exciting
opportunities. Even though it involves a lot of bother, it

may not be particularly stressful. However, in someone seventy or eighty years old, a simple move can be extremely stressful. It may mean leaving behind a lifetime of relationships and mementos. And it often does not mean a new, exciting opportunity but rather a move to what the older person may see as a more restrictive setting, whether it is a smaller apartment, a room in a relative's house, or an institution.

Often relatives and younger friends may be surprised and hurt that an older person is obviously disturbed by a move, is having trouble sleeping, and is showing other signs of stress when they have worked so hard to take care of all the physical details to make the move as smooth as possible. One has to remember that there is a great deal more involved in the move than the physical details and that a stressful reaction, including insomnia, is not unusual.

In terms of treatment, it is useful to have people to talk with when there is a period of stress. Sometimes friends and relatives will do; sometimes a counselor or therapist is helpful. And in terms of the sleep problem itself, the most important thing is to realize that it is an expectable part of a stress reaction, that it will pass with time, and that it does not require vigorous treatment measures. Sleeping medication is generally not needed. If it is prescribed, there should be a clear understanding between the doctor and patient that the medication will be used in relatively small amounts and that it will be stopped after a few weeks. A great danger is overreacting to stress as though it were a serious disease and taking various powerful medications that may be difficult to discontinue later—a situation in which the cure is worse than the disease.

AROUSAL AND CONDITIONING FACTORS

A disorder officially called persistent psychophysiological insomnia refers to a group of related

conditions that are fairly common but not totally understood. The insomnia is long-term—sometimes characterized by difficulty falling asleep, sometimes by
waking up during the night, but always by some sort of
increased body arousal at night. This insomnia usually
has no clear-cut time of onset; it lasts for years and has
become in some sense a habit. There is no total agreement as to causes or treatment, but a number of factors
appear to be important. Some people with persistent
insomnia are especially sensitive to any noise or disturbance. In these cases, sleeping in a very quiet, dark
room and using earplugs and eye shields if needed can
be a tremendous help. Sometimes the body somatizes
tension, which means that tensions, or concerns, are
somehow taken up by the muscles and the rest of the
body. When this happens at night, it produces difficulty in getting to sleep or difficulty in getting back to
sleep after an awakening. In this case, programs in
muscular relaxation, meditation, and biofeedback, as
well as supportive psychotherapy, can be of help.

Sometimes the habit aspects of the insomnia are
very strong. Most of us associate our beds with sleep.
When we "hit the bed," we are already partly asleep
because we know that bed is a place where we sleep. In
people who have this long-term psychophysiological
insomnia, the opposite association is established. These
people—for one reason or another, perhaps early sensitivity, perhaps traumatic events—have associated bed
with a painful and difficult place, where they worry or
toss and turn and do not fall asleep. For them, the
simple act of getting into bed sets up the wrong kind of
conditioned response. They feel they are not going to
be able to sleep, they become upset, their muscles become tense, and a vicious circle is set up (see figure 15).

People who react this way often note that they
sleep better when they are away from home. Peter

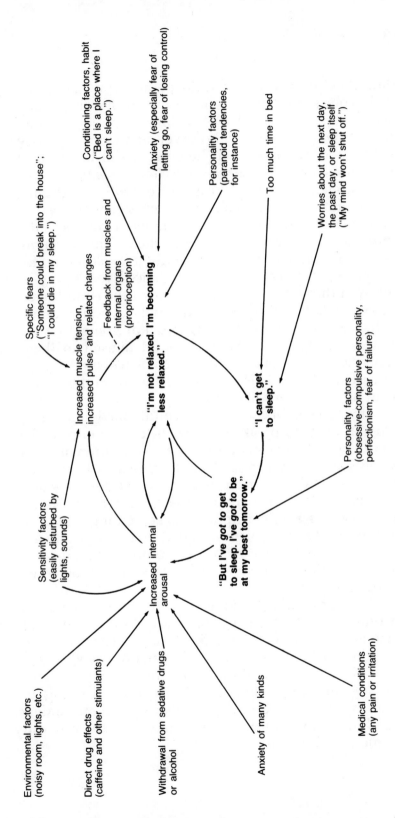

Figure 15. Vicious circles in psychophysiological insomnia

Hauri, a sleep researcher at Dartmouth University, describes one such patient, who claimed he hardly got any sleep in his own bed. He sometimes slept better when he was away from home, however, and in fact, the one really good night of sleep he could recall in the past years occurred when he was on a climbing expedition in the mountains. His party was unexpectedly caught in a storm, and they had to sleep in their sleeping bags, in hammocks strung from spikes hammered into the cliffs, with the wind howling all about them. This certainly sounds like an uncomfortable situation for sleep, but for this particular person, the circumstances were so different from those of his bed at home that the conditioned reflex did not take place. He did not have the notion, "Ah, now I'm going to bed, and I'm going to have trouble sleeping." Rather, he found himself in these very unusual conditions with which he had little experience. This allowed his body's tiredness simply to take over, and he "slept like a baby."

If you have this habitual, or conditioned, insomnia, you can learn to break the habit or put an end to the conditioning. You can do this by making sure your bed is only a place where you sleep. Don't watch TV or read in bed. If you've been in bed five or ten minutes and find that instead of becoming sleepy, you're becoming more wide awake, get up and do something else until you're really tired. This is tough at first, but eventually it works. Sometimes it helps to start off with a different bed in a different room—a bed without any insomnia association.

In a broad sense, long-term psychophysiological insomnia is a sleeplessness maintained by a number of vicious circles (see figure 15). Treatment can involve breaking these patterns in one of many ways, as we have discussed. When these measures are insufficient, therapy and counseling should be tried. Getting to know one's fears, becoming familiar with them, understanding them, and working them out in therapy can frequently be helpful.

DEPRESSION

Major affective disorder, or serious depression, is yet another common cause of insomnia in older persons. Poor sleep, especially a pattern of awaking frequently during the night or in the early morning, can often be the first symptom of severe depression.

Depression-related insomnia is *not* lifelong or long-standing. The onset is often insidious—there is no definite starting point—but sleeping troubles seem to become worse over a period of two, three, or four months. The difficulty is most often not in falling asleep but rather in remaining asleep—many awakenings, especially in the second half of the night, and early morning awakening with inability to fall back to sleep—which leads to feeling generally unable to function the next morning. In some cases, oversleeping—sleeping longer than usual—can be a sign of depression as well, but this is far less common in older persons.

If you find yourself developing this kind of sleep pattern, it is worth asking yourself whether you have other symptoms of a major depression, such as loss of energy, loss of appetite, loss of weight, and a general loss of interest in things that previously interested you. These are important symptoms that may indicate severe depression that may require treatment. The feelings most commonly thought of as occurring with depression are feelings of hopelessness, helplessness, guilt, and worthlessness—"What good am I to anyone? You would all be better off if I were dead." There is a general feeling of being "down," sometimes even suicidal.

When these feelings accompany the bodily symptoms discussed earlier, there is a full-blown major depression. You may want to use the depression scale on pages 79–80 to help decide whether you or someone you know is becoming severely depressed. (A score of eleven or above indicates that you may need professional help.)

A great deal of hope exists for this kind of depression. It is not the end of the world, though the patient often thinks she—it is more often she than he—is going downhill, is simply dying, and might as well end it all. Actually, it is not a question of going downhill. It is a matter of a self-limited illness, which usually gets better by itself in six to twelve months but can improve faster with the proper medication and supportive therapy. Treatment exists, and with treatment or, if one waits long enough, even without specific treatment, one will return to normal. You are not going downhill or dying, though you may feel you are. People who go through a severe depression and then improve and recover find themselves about where they were before the depression. They may be a few months older but otherwise are in just as good shape and just as capable of functioning in all ways as they were before.

Catherine T. was an active, hardworking social worker, age sixty-four, who had been living alone for the six years since her divorce. She was a bright woman, often very sharp and critical of others. Her children and their families, who did not live far away, knew that she was sometimes moody and liked to be left alone. Although they were all on good terms, they saw each other only every two months or so.

Catherine had always slept well but developed severe insomnia one spring. She would fall asleep all right but awake after two or three hours and either not fall back to sleep at all or doze off and on for a few hours, getting little good sleep. She felt miserable and tired in the mornings. When, after a few weeks, the situation had not improved, she consulted her internist. He prescribed a sleeping pill, which helped very little. Her sleep became worse and worse.

Over the next weeks, she began eating less and losing weight and gradually lost interest in most of her activities—even in her work, which she had always loved. When she saw her children, she seemed more cranky than usual and just wanted to be left alone. She told her daughter that she was just getting old, and she guessed she was "over the hill." She told her son that she had become a worthless old woman; she said she knew that he didn't care for her anymore and wanted her to die anyway, and she figured she might as well be dead. She insinuated that he would be glad when she died and that he was hoping she would die soon so he could inherit her money. The children found this behavior distressing and found it difficult to spend time with her; they decided they had better stay out of her way for a time.

Catherine also complained a lot and was curt with people at work. Her co-workers were relieved when she decided to take sick leave. No one saw her for a few weeks until a woman neighbor in her apartment building became quite worried when Catherine, who usually took good care of herself, came out in the hallway one day looking haggard, dirty, and disheveled and asked the neighbor whether she could borrow a few sleeping pills. The neighbor was sufficiently alarmed to call a local hospital emergency room. The emergency room in turn called the local mental health center, who referred this case to their crisis-intervention team. A member of the team came to Catherine's apartment with a police officer that evening. They found a dirty, unswept apartment filled with trash and dirty dishes. Catherine was lying on the bed apparently asleep; but the noise of their entry didn't wake her, and they were unable to arouse her. When they found an empty bottle of sleeping pills in the bathroom, they rushed her to the hospital.

Fortunately, they arrived in time. Catherine recovered from the overdose within two days and was moved to a psychiatric unit, where a diagnosis of depression was made.

Catherine was treated with antidepressant medication and supportive psychotherapy. She made a complete recovery in two months and shortly thereafter was back at work and back on fairly good terms with her family. Catherine's life was actually better than before because she and her children met several times with the psychiatric staff and were able to air some of their mutual concerns. Catherine came to realize that her pride and her need to be totally self-sufficient had kept her from seeing as much of her children as she would have liked. After her illness, they all got together more and with less tension than before.

Major depression is a common illness in the population and even more common in older persons. In anyone with serious insomnia that is not long-standing but is becoming increasingly severe over a period of weeks or months, depression should at least be considered as a possible diagnosis.

If you know an older person with some of these symptoms, it is worthwhile to get help for that person. You may not only be helping treat an illness but also be saving a life, for suicide attempts are frequently made by depressed persons. When we think of tragic suicides, we usually think of a young person; we read about increasing suicides among teenagers. These deaths stand out because they are often dramatic and unexpected and because there are so few other causes of death among teenagers. However, the actual suicide rate rises with each decade of age. We do not hear so much about this high suicide rate because it is somewhat hidden by other causes of death—heart disease, cancer, and so on—which are even more frequent in older age. Suicide is obviously a serious problem, and a person considering suicide is usually, though perhaps not always, a person who is depressed, who needs help, and who will feel better in a few months if the proper help is obtained. With that help, many suicides can be prevented. If you know someone who is thinking or talking about suicide, *assume* that the person is depressed and needs help. An older person who is talking about being useless and burdensome and mentions suicide is very likely suffering from depression, and you will be doing him or her a great favor by paying attention and getting some help.

DEPRESSION SCALE—MATURE ADULTS

Choose the best answer for how you felt
over the past week.

1. Are you basically satisfied with your life?   Yes/No

2. Have you dropped many of your activities and
   interests?   Yes/No

3. Do you feel that your life is empty?   Yes/No

4. Do you often get bored?   Yes/No

5. Are you hopeful about the future?   Yes/No

6. Are you bothered by thoughts you can't get
   out of your head?   Yes/No

7. Are you in good spirits most of the time?   Yes/No

8. Are you afraid that something bad is going to
   happen to you?   Yes/No

9. Do you feel happy most of the time?   Yes/No

10. Do you often feel helpless?   Yes/No

11. Do you often get restless and fidgety?   Yes/No

12. Do you prefer to stay at home rather than go
    out and do new things?   Yes/No

13. Do you frequently worry about the future?   Yes/No

14. Do you feel you have more problems with
    memory than most?   Yes/No

15. Do you think it is wonderful to be alive now?   Yes/No

16. Do you often feel downhearted and blue?   Yes/No

17. Do you feel pretty worthless the way you are
    now?   Yes/No

18. Do you worry a lot about the past?   Yes/No

19. Do you find life very exciting?   Yes/No

20. Is it hard for you to get started on new
    projects?   Yes/No

Continued on next page

DEPRESSION SCALE—*Continued*

21. Do you feel full of energy?   Yes/No

22. Do you feel that your situation is hopeless?   Yes/No

23. Do you think that most people are better off
    than you are?   Yes/No

24. Do you frequently get upset over little things?   Yes/No

25. Do you frequently feel like crying?   Yes/No

26. Do you have trouble concentrating?   Yes/No

27. Do you enjoy getting up in the morning?   Yes/No

28. Do you prefer to avoid social gatherings?   Yes/No

29. Is it easy for you to make decisions?   Yes/No

30. Is your mind as clear as it used to be?   Yes/No

Scoring Key

Score 1 point for a No   to questions 1, 5, 7, 9, 15, 19, 21, 27,
                         29, and 30.

Score 1 point for a Yes to questions 2, 3, 4, 6, 8, 10, 11, 12,
                         13, 14, 16, 17, 18, 20, 22, 23, 24, 25,
                         26, and 28.

A score of 11 or more is an indicator that you may be clinically
depressed. This is not a substitute for a diagnosis by a
physician. However, you may want to consult a psychiatrist or
other health professional if you have a score of over 11 points
on this questionnaire.

Source: Jerome A. Yesavage, M.D., et al., "Development and Validation
of a Geriatric Depression Scale: A Preliminary Report," *Journal of
Psychiatric Research* 17, no. 1 (1983): 41.

GUILT OR REMORSE

Guilt—not legal guilt but the emotion of remorse, feeling one has hurt someone unnecessarily—is an important human emotion given its due by playwrights and novelists but often buried by doctors and even psychiatrists as only a possible symptom of depression. Guilt, however, plays a larger role; it is prominent in many people who are not depressed and is among the psychological factors that can play a role in insomnia. We are all aware of this when we stop to think of it. Shakespeare's Macbeth may have put it best on contemplating his inability to sleep after his murder of the king of Scotland: "Macbeth does murder sleep."

   In the insomnia of older persons, in fact, guilt or remorse about actions in the past may play a larger role than does anxiety about the future, which is a common cause of not falling asleep in the young.

   Most of us are not Macbeths—slayers of kings—but we are all capable of guilt and remorse that may take many subtle forms. Quite frequently, when someone close to us has died, we find ourselves examining the relationship with that person in various ways; the ambivalent aspects of the relationship then emerge. We sense, often not quite consciously, that we have angry feelings toward the deceased person; or we feel that we did not treat him or her as well as we should have. We wish we had told the person about some of the good feelings; now it is too late . . . and so on. These feelings are often deep and gnawing; they form part of the process of mourning or mild depression that follows most deaths. This sort of guilt and remorse is not limited to the elderly, but as we get older, more people close to us are dying or dead, and more of our time and energy is devoted to thinking about this. These feelings are worth exploring in any way possible. The guilt that remains unconscious or half-conscious for long periods, whether or not it is part of a full-blown depression, often appears to be involved in long-term insomnia.

SLEEPING PILLS

In the past sleeping pills have been the most common treatment for insomnia—one that has been overused. Diagnosing a specific problem and then treating that problem is the best approach. A sleeping pill merely treats the symptom. Sleeping pills do have a use, but one must be aware of their limits—the drawbacks as well as the advantages of use.

Sleeping pills are useful in a short-term situation involving a known trauma or stress that will produce insomnia—at the time of a surgical operation, for example. They can also be helpful at times of nonsurgical medical stress stemming from an acute arthritic inflammation, for instance, that despite the use of proper analgesics still is uncomfortable enough to prevent sleep for a number of days. Sleeping pills may be useful also for brief periods with conditions such as transient psychophysiological insomnia.

In all these situations the doctor and patient should be aware that there is likely to be a difficult period after withdrawal of sleeping medication. Even someone who has no previous insomnia may have a few days—or sometimes more—of insomnia after withdrawing from sleeping pills. Someone who has previously had insomnia may have a longer-term problem. You and your physician should be aware of this during the period of withdrawal insomnia. You should not decide that since you are having insomnia, you need to return to sleeping pills; if you do, you may find yourself taking them for the rest of your life.

Only occasionally should sleeping pills be prescribed on a long-term basis—for months or years. Some people do require long-term sleeping medication, either because they have an unusual chemical constitution or some ingrained psychological pattern that is so strong that it resists any alteration. I usually consider long-term sleeping medication as a last resort, to be used very rarely and only when there is severe long-term insomnia that has not responded to an attempt at diagnosis and specific treatment.

The reason most sleep disorders specialists are so careful about using sleep medication is that traditionally these sleep medications have had many problems and side effects associated with them. Many sleeping medications are respiratory depressants; most are physically and/or psychologically addictive; most have serious interactions with alcohol or sometimes with other medications that can make specific conditions such as sleep apnea worse; and, in general, they alter laboratory-recorded sleep patterns severely by reducing deep, slow-wave sleep and REM sleep, the two stages of sleep we think may be the most essential and restorative.

The more recently developed sleeping pills are in the group called the benzodiazepines. These include, for instance, flurazepam (Dalmane), temazepam (Restoril), and triazolam (Halcion). These are safer than the older sleeping pills, since they produce much less respiratory depression, but they still cause the other problems. The benzodiazepines sometimes produce problems, especially in older persons, because their effect builds up over many days; they may help insomnia while producing a disturbing degree of daytime sleepiness.

In situations where some sleep medication is required, especially in older persons, there are several alternatives to the use of the standard sleeping pills. One alternative is the group of antihistamines, the standard medications that show up in over-the-counter cold capsules and produce drowsiness. These are not powerful, but they do have some sleep-inducing effect and are safe for most people. Another alternative is the amino acid tryptophan, which was already mentioned briefly. This is a food substance and at the moment is classified only as a food, not as a medication, by the Food and Drug Administration; however, a great deal of research indicates that it does improve sleep. It reduces the time it takes to fall asleep and reduces the time spent awake to some extent as well. Since it is a food substance, it should at least be relatively safe. Since even these two safer alternatives to traditional sleeping pills can possibly interact with other medication, it is best to consult your physician before taking them.

◀ 7 ▶

Hypersomnolence

If you are feeling more and more tired in the daytime, and perhaps falling asleep when you don't want to, you may have a serious problem that requires help. Your complaint is called excessive daytime sleepiness (EDS). If you actually are sleeping a great many more hours than normal, say twelve to sixteen hours per each twenty-four-hour period, you have hypersomnia, a much rarer complaint than EDS. The two complaints EDS and hypersomnia are included under the term *hypersomnolence*. Hypersomnolence is a symptom, as insomnia is, with many distinct causes. Of course, the two symptoms are sometimes related. If you have severe insomnia, you may also complain of daytime sleepiness because you are not getting enough sleep.

Some persons, as they get older, tend to doze more and sometimes sleep more in the daytime. If you have this problem, don't assume that you're simply "getting old" or "going downhill." Daytime dozing should not occur to a major extent until one is at least in one's seventies or eighties. If you are fifty-five or sixty-five and are becoming very tired in the daytime, you definitely should not assume that it is a matter of aging. And even if you or a loved one is eighty, it is best not to conclude that the sleepiness is simply due to aging and that nothing can be done about it—especially if the sleepiness has come on rapidly in a period of days, weeks, or months rather than very gradually over a period of years. In fact, there are a considerable number of medical and psychological conditions that can produce daytime sleepiness, and many of these conditions are quite easy to treat or to change.

While there may be some doctors who automatically treat the symptom insomnia with a sleeping pill, neglecting to seek an underlying cause, I doubt that there are any who would automatically treat excessive daytime sleepiness with a stimulant: "Oh, you're feeling tired, and you sleep a lot in the daytime? Here, have some amphetamines." Some people, however, do exactly this to themselves. A woman who found she was becoming gradually more tired in the daytime, without thinking much about it, gradually increased her use of coffee to keep herself awake. It was only after a few months when she was feeling jittery and "jazzed up" every evening that she suddenly realized she had increased her coffee consumption gradually from three cups to over fifteen cups a day. At that point, she finally decided she had better look into why she needed so much coffee in the daytime. It turned out that her daytime fatigue was caused by a treatable medical condition—nocturnal myoclonus.

MEDICAL CAUSES FOR
HYPERSOMNOLENCE

As is the case with insomnia, there are many medical causes for daytime sleepiness. The following discussion will give you some idea of whether you may have a particular medical condition; however, a specialist and special tests are generally required to determine the exact diagnosis and the best treatment. Fortunately most of the medical causes for daytime sleepiness are treatable.

Sleep Apnea

Although sleep apnea is a cause of insomnia, it is more often a cause of daytime sleepiness; sometimes it produces both symptoms.

The word *apnea* means "not breathing" or "no breathing," and indeed sleep apnea refers to not breathing during sleep. Our breathing apparatus is so much a part of us—we simply expect it to continue no matter what else we do—that the idea of not breathing seems strange to us, and yet this is exactly what happens to many people. The control of respiration is considerably different during sleep than it is during wakefulness. Recordings demonstrate that in some people, airflow (air entering or leaving the nose or mouth) simply stops—not just a few times but in severe cases several hundred times during the night. Luckily, reflex mechanisms wake us up when oxygen levels become too low or carbon dioxide levels too high, so breathing stops usually for only ten to thirty seconds. An arousal quickly follows, during which the person starts to breathe again.

The mechanisms producing sleep apnea are complex, but basically there are two major ways that airflow can stop. With central sleep apnea, the neurons of the central nervous system responsible for sending out impulses to the respiratory muscles simply do not function or do not function adequately. Central sleep apnea is seen in infants in whom the mechanisms in the brain responsible for regulating sleep have not yet developed fully. It is seen in adults who have had neurological disorders—especially those affecting the brain stem, such as polio—and it occurs for unknown reasons in some older people who have not had any illness.

In obstructive sleep apnea the breathing muscles in the diaphragm and chest continue to function, but something blocks the flow of air through the neck. Sometimes this is simply fatty tissue in someone who is overweight; sometimes the blockage involves a tumor or other disease condition in the throat. But often the blockage seems to be caused by an improper opening of the posterior pharynx (back of the throat) so that air does not get through properly with each breath. In this last instance, obstructive and central apnea are not so different, since neuromuscular problems affecting nerve impulses to the throat muscles can produce an obstruction of the throat and, thus, obstructive apnea.

Recordings at a sleep center often reveal mixed sleep apnea—partly obstructive and partly central apnea. In these cases, the primary problem is usually obstructive apnea; the brain, when it senses an obstruction, appears to react by shutting off breathing impulses. All types of apnea become more prevalent in our fifties and sixties, and about one-fourth of us have some degree of apnea by the time we reach seventy. One study just completed by Dr. Sonia Ancoli-Israel and co-workers in San Diego involved all-night sleep recordings in 427 randomly selected persons over sixty-five. The average age of those studied was seventy-two. In this group, 24 percent had a significant degree of sleep apnea. Most of these subjects were not complaining of any sleep problems and did not require immediate treatment; however, it is very common for these conditions to worsen gradually, so many of these people may eventually complain of poor sleep or excessive daytime sleepiness (EDS) in the next few years.

If untreated, severe sleep apnea can be dangerous. First of all, because of the poor sleep or the lack of oxygen at night, the apnea sufferer is unusually sleepy in the daytime and may, for example, fall asleep while driving or while operating dangerous machinery. Occasionally, sleep apnea seems to produce poor mental functioning or even something resembling dementia, presumably due to lack of sufficient oxygen to the brain. However, most often this is a temporary condition related to excessive tiredness, and the mental functioning improves once the apnea is treated. In addition, untreated sleep apnea can lead to pulmonary problems, cardiac problems (enlargement of the heart and cardiac arrhythmias), and increased blood pressure. All of these are thought to result from the loss of oxygen during the night, which forces the heart to work harder and thickens the blood vessel walls.

It is worth keeping in mind that increasing weight, sleep apnea, and increasing blood pressure often go together. There are complicated relationships between these three conditions. One of the more common patterns is that one first gains weight—for whatever reason. The weight gain brings on sleep apnea—chiefly obstructive apnea—or perhaps makes worse a case of apnea that was not previously producing any problems. The sleep apnea then gradually, over a period of months and years, brings on higher blood pressure, and high blood pressure, as we know, can lead to such serious conditions as heart attack and stroke.

Sometimes the situation can become more complicated. Weight gain can produce sleep apnea or increase its severity, but the converse can also occur: A person developing sleep apnea—as a gradual change with age or for any other reason—will become more and more tired, and, thus, less active in the daytime. If food consumption doesn't change, this will lead to weight gain, and the weight gain will make the apnea worse. Then together these two will eventually lead to increased blood pressure. I emphasize this relationship because physicians have only recently begun to understand it, and many are still not aware of it.

Physicians who see someone with high blood pressure will tend to prescribe medication and/or a low-salt diet; they most often call the condition essential hypertension (high blood pressure with no known cause) and seldom think to examine the patient for sleep apnea. A recent study, conducted by Dr. Anthony Kales in Hershey, Pennsylvania, examined fifty middle-aged people chosen simply because their blood pressure was in the range usually called hypertensive. They were not chosen on the basis of any sleep problems. Each of these men and women's sleep was recorded in the sleep laboratory; it turned out that one-third had a significant degree of sleep apnea.

It is important to know this, since it is in a sense a hopeful sign. Hypertension is often thought of as a condition that becomes more common with age, is bound to become worse, and seldom improves, though it can be controlled to some extent with medication. However, it now turns out that there are many cases in which hypertension is secondary to sleep apnea. When the sleep apnea is properly treated, the blood pressure not only stops increasing but often actually decreases toward normal levels.

Apnea is often, but not always, associated with snoring at night. In deciding whether someone has apnea, it is very important to talk not only with the sufferer but also with the spouse, bedmate, or room-mate. An apnea sufferer may simply notice daytime tiredness and may say, "I guess I sleep all right at night. I seem to get eight hours a night." However, the wife (the majority of apnea patients are men) may have a very different story: "He spends eight hours in bed, but I don't think he gets much good sleep. He's a very restless sleeper. He snores so heavily it drives everyone away. He gasps and chokes sometimes. Sometimes his snoring will suddenly stop, and he won't breathe at all for a while. He gets me worried."

If apnea is strongly suspected because of symptoms like these, one should definitely have a polysomnogram (an all-night sleep study) at a sleep disorders center. This is the only way that the diagnosis can be made definite and the severity of the apnea can be established so that proper treatment can be initiated.

A person with sleep apnea obtains very little continuous sleep. The patient is quite unaware of the poor sleep at night but may be aware of the daytime sleepiness. He is worried because he is falling asleep at work, or at a party. One patient who turned out to have typical apnea told me, "I can't understand it. I sleep fine at night. In fact, I sometimes spend nine or ten hours asleep. But in the past year or two I have been falling asleep in the damnedest places. I fell asleep at a business conference three or four times. I fall asleep having dinner with my wife and friends, and I am really worried because the other day I started to fall asleep at the wheel and drove right off the highway before I caught myself."

We now often speak of "the apneas" or "respiratory impairments," since there are several other conditions related to sleep apnea. One such condition is hypopnea, in which breathing slows but does not actually stop. With another condition, alveolar hypoventilation, air does pass through the throat but because of thickening in the lung tissues does not properly reach the membranes of the small alveoli in the lungs, where oxygen is absorbed.

With proper medical help, sleep apnea is definitely a treatable condition. The treatment is a complicated issue that is best handled by a sleep disorders expert, since effective treatment depends on the type and severity of the condition, and this can be best determined by an expert. Treatment can include weight loss, gadgets that make it difficult for a patient to sleep on his or her back, several different medications, continuous positive airway pressure (a pump device that pushes air in through a mask all night), and surgical procedures.

I hope all older persons will consider sleep apnea and other conditions discussed here when assessing their sleep problems and will not simply attribute daytime sleepiness to old age or "going downhill." I have seen several men and women who were becoming more and more sleepy in the daytime, could figure out no reason for it, and assumed that this was simply part of becoming old. This "diagnosis" appeared to them to be confirmed by the fact that they had some memory loss and seemed to get confused easily in the daytime. It turned out that *all* these symptoms were secondary to sleep apnea. When the apnea was treated, they slept better at night, as reported by their spouses and as verified by sleep recordings. They were less sleepy in the daytime and, much to their surprise, they felt better, thought better, became less forgetful, and found that they were not going downhill after all.

Nocturnal Myoclonus
Periodic movements during sleep (nocturnal myoclonus) is a common condition that is not yet well understood. However, it has definitely been shown to be more common in older persons than in younger ones. *Myoclonus* refers to repeated jerking movements of the muscles, most often the leg muscles but sometimes the arm muscles and others as well. A person who has severe myoclonus seems to be kicking and twitching all night long. Sometimes this is obvious to a bedmate, but it is often not noticed by the person with the problem. This condition is perhaps a bit more prevalent among women than among men. Sometimes, as with apnea, the only complaint is excessive daytime sleepiness—feeling tired all day or not feeling rested in the morning. More often, the person will be aware of the arousals following these muscle jerks and will complain of insomnia. The diagnosis and treatment of myoclonus has already been discussed in chapter 5, "Insomnia: Medical Causes."

Narcolepsy
A strange but by now quite well-studied condition, narcolepsy consists primarily of attacks of irresistible sleepiness in the daytime. The patient typically falls asleep suddenly while watching TV or sitting at a meeting. In severe cases, attacks of sleep occur while en-

gaged in important activity, such as when driving or even while making love.

Associated symptoms—including cataplexy, hypnogogic hallucinations, and sleep paralysis—help make the diagnosis of narcolepsy, though no one of them is always present. Cataplexy is characterized by sudden loss of muscle tone and collapse (or partial collapse) during wakefulness. Sometimes the patient remains conscious; sometimes there is a brief loss of consciousness associated with the experience of dreaming. A strong emotion such as anger sometimes precipitates an attack of cataplexy. Hypnogogic hallucinations occur while falling asleep or occasionally while waking up; the patient has a kind of hallucination in which he or she sees someone else in the room or hears someone calling his or her name. But the hallucination passes very quickly, and the patient is then sure that no one was really there. Sleep paralysis is a condition in which one is "half awake" in the sense of the mind being awake but the muscles refusing to move. Almost everyone has occasionally had a brief episode; if it continues for more than a few seconds, it may be a sign of narcolepsy. In any case, someone who has attacks of irresistible sleep with one or more of these other symptoms is quite likely to have narcolepsy, though there are some other questions one must ask as well.

If narcolepsy is suspected, one must have a recording made at a sleep disorders center or by a neurologist at a hospital to confirm the diagnosis. The most reliable confirmation can be obtained by what is called a Multiple Sleep Latency Test (MSLT), in which the person is given four or five opportunities to fall asleep during the daytime and twenty-minute recordings are made. Someone with narcolepsy not only falls asleep quickly but falls quickly into rapid eye movement (REM) sleep. A nighttime recording may sometimes be useful as well; it will help rule out other causes of daytime sleepiness, such as apnea and myoclonus.

Narcolepsy runs in families to a certain extent. It is

not specifically a disease of older persons. In fact, older persons will be glad to hear that narcolepsy very seldom begins after age thirty or forty. Most often, it begins around age fifteen or twenty and is thereafter a lifelong condition. However, it still cannot be ruled out in older persons because many patients are not aware that they have had narcolepsy for many years. They may have found themselves falling asleep in class or at meetings but explained it away as a response to lack of sleep or to dull work. They fought off sleep attacks often by using very large amounts of coffee or tea and never realized that they may have had an actual illness until years later.

A number of treatments for narcolepsy are available, and more and better treatments should be available soon based on the high level of current research. At the moment, treatment usually consists of using stimulant medication such as amphetamines or methylphenidate (Ritalin) in the daytime. In some cases, especially when cataplexy is present, other medications are required and are useful. The disturbing "accessory symptoms" such as cataplexy and sleep paralysis almost always improve or cease with proper medication. In some cases, narcolepsy can be treated without medication by carefully spacing naps during the day to relieve the excessive sleepiness, since one characteristic of narcolepsy is that short daytime sleep periods are refreshing, and the person feels better able to function after having one.

Dementia and Alzheimer's Disease

Dementia, the loss of mental powers, is something that we all fear for ourselves as well as for our older relatives. The most common cause of dementia in older persons is Alzheimer's disease. Dementia, including Alzheimer's disease, does eventually lead to dozing and sleeping in the daytime. However, it is not in the least true that if one sleeps or dozes in the daytime, one should think of dementia as a probable cause. In fact, by the time dementia progresses to the point where there is a great deal of daytime sleep, serious mental problems have almost certainly been obvious for some time.

Alzheimer's disease is a formidable problem because its exact causes and mechanisms are as yet not known, and there is no definite treatment for it. The disease involves the gradual loss of memory, ability to think and to recognize people and objects, and eventually ability to communicate with others and to take care of oneself. This course of deterioration is now fairly well established. Fortunately, we now know that relatively few older persons actually develop this disease. Alzheimer's is not something that simply comes with age but is a specific disease that afflicts perhaps 5 percent of older people. It is quite possible that even when many symptoms of dementia are present, other conditions—and, in fact, treatable conditions—may be responsible for those symptoms.

Within this general warning not to accept the diagnosis of Alzheimer's disease too quickly, I would like to reiterate the point that sleep problems are not especially prominent among its symptoms. A person who does have Alzheimer's may indeed have disturbed sleep-wake patterns as part of the overall picture (both insomnia and hypersomnolence may occur), but a sleep problem—a serious complaint of insomnia or of daytime sleepiness or, for that matter, of nightmares, night terrors, and so on—is very seldom the chief concern. Thus, when an older person complains of a serious sleep disorder, it is in some sense a good sign. A person who may have some of the characteristics of Alzheimer's disease—for example, poor memory or lowered performance at work—but who also complains of daytime sleepiness and/or serious insomnia may quite possibly have a depression or sleep apnea rather than Alzheimer's disease.

Medication

Chemical substances—prescribed medications, nonprescribed medications, and alcohol—are a common cause of daytime sleepiness, especially in the elderly. There are a large variety of medications that can produce daytime sleepiness as a side effect. If you have been keeping a record of all the medication you have been taking (see the chart on pages 62-63), you should be able to determine whether the sleepiness is related to the onset of the medication, or perhaps to an increased dosage. Remember that sleepiness may not come on like a sledgehammer the day after you start new medication, though this sometimes happens. When it does, the connection is quite obvious. But there are other possibilities. One is the experience of some daytime tiredness that is fairly severe for a few days after starting medication but that then becomes less and less severe with time. This probably means that you had an initial side effect that has worn off, and it may be all right to continue taking the medication. On the other hand, you may find in looking at the chart that the tiredness has gradually built up over a period of several weeks after the time you started (or increased) the medication. This is an indication that the medication may be building up in your body and that your doctor should consider reducing the medication, stopping it, or changing to something else.

Among the medications that can cause daytime sleepiness are, first of all, the sleeping pills and tranquilizers. Many physicians do not realize that older persons store and metabolize these medications differently and that the same dose of medication may often have a much greater effect in an older person than in a younger one. Thus, when a physician prescribes a typical dose of sleeping pill—for example, thirty milligrams of flurazepam (Dalmane) to be taken at bedtime—it will indeed produce sleep at night, but often, you, the older person, will note that you are becoming more and more tired in the daytime. This is because the level of medication gradually builds up in the body. After a week or two of Dalmane, you may have as much in your blood in the daytime as you need at night to put you to sleep. If you keep taking large doses of sleeping pills, you will notice other symptoms besides daytime sleepiness. These may include problems in muscular coordination—difficulty in holding things or a tendency to fall—disorientation, and even confusion or delirium.

In these situations, the treatment is relatively simple—reduce the dose, discontinue the medication, or change the medication. Some physicians are under the impression that the so-called short-acting sleeping pills—the most common ones used now are temazepam (Restoril) and triazolam (Halcion)—are much safer and cannot produce these long-term daytime effects. Unfortunately, however, this is not always the case. In older persons, the effects may be longer lasting than expected; even a so-called short-acting sleeping pill can produce effects during the day. And it may sometimes take a week or several weeks for such effects to show up. Frequently used tranquilizers such as diazepam (Valium), chlordiazepoxide (Librium), chlorazepate (Tranxene), and lorazepam (Ativan) are in the same class (benzodiazepines) as the sleeping pills mentioned, and they can also produce a gradual buildup of daytime sleepiness.

The older sleeping pills, especially the barbiturates, which indeed were called sedatives and often used in the daytime, will produce daytime sleepiness—sometimes they are meant to do exactly this—but one must be careful about the dose. One reason these pills are not used as much now is that they can be quite dangerous. Used in appropriate doses, they have a calming, or sedative, effect, but the problem is that a dose not very much larger will produce unwanted daytime sleepiness, and a dose not very much larger than that may actually produce respiratory depression and states of coma or occasionally death. Thus, it is worth keeping in mind that all sleeping pills and tranquilizers can produce daytime sleepiness and these other dangerous side effects and can do it more easily in older persons than in younger ones because of differences in metabolism and sensitivity.

Many other medications not considered tranquilizers or sleeping pills may produce tiredness or sleepiness as a side effect. This is true of many medications taken for high blood pressure, some cardiac medications, antihistamines taken for allergies or colds, and medications taken as antidepressants and as antipsychotics.

A very different group of medications, the stimulants, can also, in a particular context, produce sleepiness. The stimulants include amphetamines (Benzedrine, Dexedrine), methylphenidate (Ritalin), cocaine and related street drugs, and caffeine. The stimulant medications, which normally make one especially alert or awake during use, can produce excessive sleepiness upon withdrawal. Someone who has been taking amphetamines for a long time as a treatment for narcolepsy, let us say, or as an old-fashioned treatment for obesity (they are now seldom used in this way) or has been taking a tremendous amount of caffeine and suddenly stops will almost certainly have a period of sleeping more than usual or of daytime somnolence. This effect is to be expected, and no treatment is necessary except the passage of time.

Withdrawal from stimulants is not a common cause for sleepiness in older persons but can be very dramatic and frightening when it occurs. One fifty-five-year-old woman who was taking amphetamines for obesity had, on her own, gradually increased the dose to quite high levels over a period of two years; realizing she had become addicted, she suddenly stopped taking them. This woman slept almost twenty hours in each twenty-four-hour period during the following week before her sleep pattern gradually returned to normal.

Alcohol—With and Without Medication

Alcohol can be a major culprit in daytime sleepiness, as it is in insomnia. That someone is drinking too much should be fairly obvious, but sometimes it is not. People do not like to admit to drinking and will try to conceal the fact that they do. One rather uncommunicative man in his sixties was brought in to the sleep disorders center by his relatives because he wouldn't answer the phone, and they couldn't seem to wake him up until two or three in the afternoon. He did not think it was much of a problem. He said he was just tired and wanted to be left alone. I mentioned to him and to his family the possibility of medications or alcohol producing this sleepiness, but he denied taking alcohol or any medication. I could not find a specific cause for his sleepiness at that time, and over the following weeks the condition became increasingly worse. He started to lose weight from not eating, and finally relatives began to smell alcohol on his breath. When they finally convinced him to let them enter his apartment, they found a number of empty bottles of liquor, and it became obvious that this man, though he appeared sober when he made his few social appearances in the afternoon, had been more or less drinking himself into a stupor every night.

One should not assume that alcoholism is solely a problem of young adults. A great many older people suffer from it also. They draw less attention to themselves because they often drink at home, because they are more likely to become tired and pass out than to become violent, and perhaps because the wisdom of their years has taught them not to drive when intoxicated.

Alcohol can be especially dangerous for older persons, since they are more likely to be taking other medications, and almost all medications can interact in some way with alcohol. Perhaps the most common effect is an intensification of the sleepiness that can occur as a side effect with the use of many medications. If you are a social drinker who has become familiar with your tolerance for alcohol—you know that two glasses of wine make you a bit euphoric but won't put you to sleep—don't expect this tolerance to remain unchanged once you have started taking a tranquilizer or an antihypertensive medication. You may find yourself waking up on a couch somewhere unexpected, hours after the two innocent glasses of wine!

And alcohol can also "interact" with other conditions or illnesses. For example, some episodic sleep disorders, such as night terrors and sleepwalking, and also sleep apnea are quite frequently aggravated by alcohol. A moderate degree of sleep apnea can become severe and even life-threatening when aggravated by alcohol.

PSYCHOLOGICAL CAUSES

Daytime sleepiness does not result from psychological causes as often as it results from medical causes, but it is nonetheless important to be aware of possible psychological causes. A sleep disorders specialist can sometimes be helpful by checking to make sure that the problem is not caused by one of the medical conditions discussed. Sometimes a sleep recording can also help identify the type of psychological problem that exists.

Avoidance Reactions

Sometimes one stays in bed and sleeps just to avoid dealing with the world—to get away from things. This often happens as part of a reaction to stress or loss. When someone close has died, or the house has burned down, one reaction is to want to deny the fact, to push it away completely, and we sometimes do this by sleeping excessively for a few days or a few weeks. The process is usually not fully conscious. We don't say, "I think I'll just sleep for two weeks. Don't bother me until the fifteenth." It just happens.

Stress Reactions

Some older people, especially those over seventy, may have a stress reaction, including oversleeping, to things younger people might not consider so stressful—a move from familiar surroundings to an unfamiliar place, for example. Such a move almost always feels stressful and may result in insomnia for a while; it can also result in a period of oversleeping.

In any case, such a period of excessive sleep related to stress is not something to worry about or to treat specifically. You certainly should not take stimulant medication to reduce sleep! However, you may want to get help in dealing with your feelings about the stressful change as well as help in reorganizing your life after the change.

Depression

In older persons, severe depression is most commonly associated with difficulty in sleeping. However, in some older people who are depressed, and in many younger people, the main symptom is hypersomnia—excessive sleep—rather than lack of sleep. In these cases, the problem is seldom daytime sleepiness in the sense of suddenly falling asleep at unwanted times (as in narcolepsy) but rather sleeping longer and longer hours. People with this kind of depression need nine, ten, or twelve hours of sleep per day. In these cases, other symptoms of depression are usually present, and the depression can generally be treated with antidepressant medication and supportive psychotherapy.

MULTIPLE CAUSES FOR DAYTIME SLEEPINESS

Unfortunately, the major causes of daytime sleepiness are not always found in isolation; one person may have a number of causes for sleepiness, and the causes may reinforce one another. This can happen in an older person at times of stress or when the person is lonely or feels isolated.

One older woman was sleepy all the time and

seemed to have poor memory for recent events. The woman had lost her husband two years before. A year later she had moved to the Boston area, where she had a married child. However, she was not very close with this child or with anyone else. She lived by herself; she did not go out much and was obviously somewhat depressed, which may have been one reason for her sleepiness. However, she treated her depression with alcohol, and her drinking increased over a period of a few months. The alcohol she drank in the morning (probably to try to combat feelings of hopelessness, which are often worse in the morning) made her increasingly sleepy in the daytime but also made her increasingly sleepless at night.

She consulted a physician about her nighttime insomnia but did not tell him about her heavy alcohol intake. A sleeping pill was prescribed, which she took for several weeks while continuing the alcohol. The sleeping pill only made the situation worse. She soon was suffering from the combined effect of depression, alcohol, and sleeping medication. It was necessary for her to spend several weeks at a hospital and then at a rehabilitation center to withdraw from the alcohol and sleeping pills and to begin the process of getting involved in activities with her family and other people.

◢8◣

Sleep-Wake Schedule Disorders

The main feature characterizing a group of interesting disorders of the sleep-wake schedule is that symptoms are time related. For instance, "I try to get to bed at eleven or twelve in the evening, and I just can't get to sleep. However, I fall asleep all right if I don't go to bed until 5:00 A.M." Sometimes associated with this is the related difficulty in waking up: "I can't seem to get myself up at six or seven when I need to get up. If I let myself sleep 'til 11:00 A.M., I am fine." Such rhythm disturbances are most frequently found in younger people but can be found at times in older persons. One can understand these conditions best by thinking of jet lag, the simplest and best-known example of rhythm disturbance.

JET LAG

Consider a woman who lives on the West Coast of the United States and who always goes to bed around 11:00

P.M. and gets up at 7:00 A.M. She takes a trip to the East Coast and goes to bed at her usual time, but finds that she cannot get to sleep. She has "insomnia" because her body is still on Pacific time; her body "feels" it is only 8:00 P.M., hours before her usual bedtime. She will also experience trouble the next morning if she has to get up at 7:00 A.M. eastern standard time, which is 4:00 A.M. on the West Coast, a time when she is not used to arising. At that point, she will have "excessive daytime sleepiness." (Jet lag, of course, can be worse if you fly halfway around the world—a twelve-hour rather than a three-hour time difference.) With jet lag, the problem is obvious: One is asking one's body to go to bed and to get up at a time that seems unusual to the body, and the body rebels.

Most people adapt to jet lag within three, four, or five days. If one wishes, it is possible to reduce jet lag by starting to shift one's schedule in the appropriate direction a few days ahead of time, but most people do not find this necessary. Other treatments involving medication, exercise, and changes in diet are under investigation, but no treatment is fully established at the present time.

Jet lag is not particularly a condition of older persons, but the human body does become a little less adaptive with age, and it may take a day or two longer to adapt properly at age sixty than it did at age thirty. Thus, if you are over sixty, or if you have found jet lag to be disturbing in the past, plan your time so that you do not have a demanding schedule the first day or two after arriving in a new time zone.

IRREGULAR SCHEDULE

Jet lag is not the only such sleep-wake scheduling problem. Some people appear to suffer from jet lag without having flown across time zones! This happens to people with rapidly shifting work schedules or people who, for one reason or another, radically change their bedtimes from day to day. For instance, if you are used to sleeping from midnight to 8:00 A.M. and then take a new job or responsibility that requires you to get up at four in the morning, you may decide to go to bed at 8:00 or 9:00 P.M. In this situation, you are likely to have trouble sleeping, just as if you had jet lag, since your body is not used to going to bed at the time you demand of it.

Some people put their bodies through irregular time changes by constantly altering their schedules. They go to bed at 10:00 P.M. one night, 6:00 A.M. the next night, and 1:00 A.M. the night after that. After weeks or months of this, they may have trouble falling asleep no matter what time they go to bed, since the body is confused and does not quite know when it is supposed to feel sleepy. In this situation, one is quite likely to feel tired when one wants to be awake, and vice versa. Both daytime sleepiness and insomnia can be produced by this condition. This most frequently occurs in a young person—for instance, a graduate student working on a dissertation or someone who spends a great deal of time attending late parties. It can also occur in older persons who keep a totally irregular schedule. The treatment for such a rhythm disturbance is simple. Return to an extremely regular schedule of sleeping and waking. You can also help your body return to a stable rhythm by taking meals and exercising at regular times each day. It may take a month or more for this treatment to work, but it is generally quite successful.

DELAYED AND ADVANCED
SLEEP-PHASE SYNDROMES

Self-imposed sleep-wake disturbances occur quite often, and they are usually easy to correct. Much more rarely someone will have a true "delayed sleep-phase syndrome" or "advanced sleep-phase syndrome," in which the body's internal clock, or clocks, are out of adjustment and refuse to run on a 24-hour day. This is a situation that is just beginning to be understood. Our bodies are governed by many interdependent rhythms—endocrine rhythms, body temperature rhythms, and so on—that all run on a cycle of about 24 hours. For instance, most people's body temperature rises to a maximum every day between 2:00 P.M. and 6:00 P.M. These are called circadian rhythms (rhythms with a cycle length of about 24 hours). These rhythms are thought to be controlled by one or possibly two master clocks in the brain. In most people, these rhythms have a natural periodicity, or cycle length, of slightly over 24 hours, averaging perhaps 24.7 hours. This means that if we live in a cave, or in a laboratory with no time cues whatever, we tend to run our lives on "days" of 24.5 to 25 hours. However, under normal conditions, we use light and dark to shorten these cycles slightly and fit them into 24-hour days. We are, thus, constantly squeezing a 24.5-hour or 25-hour cycle into a 24-hour day.

A very few people are unable to shorten their 24.5-hour or 25-hour cycle to 24 hours. This may be a problem of the central nervous system, or it may occur, for instance, in someone who is blind and thus unaware of the cues provided by daylight. Such a person can develop a "free-running rhythm," tending to go to bed slightly later every night. The individual might go to bed at midnight one night, 12:40 A.M. the next night, 1:20 A.M. the night after that, and so on. This person will notice that it becomes harder and harder to go to bed at 12:00 P.M. The condition is unusual in pure form, as described, but many people may have a mild form of it and find it easier to fall asleep at a time much later than their usual bedtime.

Even more unusual is the opposite condition, advanced sleep-phase syndrome, in which the natural cycle is less than 24 hours, and the person tends to go to bed earlier every night. A number of treatments for these unusual conditions are being investigated.

SUNDOWNING

It is worth mentioning here a condition known as "sundowning," or "nocturnal wandering," which occurs frequently in older people, even though it is not directly associated with sleep.

This condition usually occurs in very old people, in persons who have had strokes, or in those who have some form of brain disease. It occurs when, due to one of these conditions, the person's brain is in a fragile state, just barely able to carry on its normal functions. In the daytime, when the living quarters are well lit and there are regular meals and other people around, the person manages all right. If one mental function isn't working perfectly, others can be used. For example, a person in a nursing home may not remember exactly how to get to the dining room at the end of the hall but can hear the noise of others eating and will then walk toward the room. If the person can see others heading for the dining room, he or she may join them, or the individual may ask someone for help.

When night falls, especially if the person is alone in a room or an apartment, many orienting cues are removed, and the person may become increasingly disoriented and unable to function, take care of himself or herself, or find his or her way around. Such a person is sometimes found wandering around, lost—hence the term *nocturnal wandering*. This is partly due to physical darkness, which removes some orienting cues, but it is worse if the older person is also left alone in the evening. This condition is not a specific illness and does not require specific treatment, except of course that the person can be helped by having more people around, having well-lit surroundings, and having more organi-

zational cues in the evening and at night. The disoriented state of sundowning can sometimes be brought
on or worsened by sleeping medications, sedatives,
tranquilizers, or alcohol, so these substances should be
used only with great care. The patient, or the person
caring for the patient, must be aware of this aspect of
medication and remain on the alert for any changes that
occur when the medication is being taken.

≡ 9 ≣

Episodic Events

It now remains to discuss the episodic events related to sleep—repeated incidents that occur irregularly and can be quite frightening. None of these conditions is specifically a problem for older persons, and they may occur at any age.

SLEEPWALKING, NIGHT TERRORS, AND ENURESIS

The best-studied episodic events are a group of three conditions that arouse the sleeper, usually within two hours of sleep onset. These are sleepwalking, night terrors, and enuresis, or bed-wetting. All three conditions are most common in childhood. It has been estimated that at least 20 percent of children at ages five to seven have at least a few episodes of sleepwalking, night terrors, or enuresis. These conditions remain fairly common in adolescence and young adulthood but then decrease steadily with age. None is very common in older persons.

Sleepwalking is obvious to an observer, though not always to the sleepwalker. Technically, one does not have to actually walk around to qualify as a sleepwalker. Some people simply stand up or sit up in bed or roll over and strike out in flailing motions without quite knowing it. Sleepwalking occurs early in the night usually and arises from stage 3 or stage 4 sleep.

Night terrors consist of episodes of screaming in terror followed by an awakening with no recall of a dream, or occasionally a recall of a single frightening image: "Something is sitting on me," or, "Something is closing in on me." In the sleep laboratory, we can show that these episodes of night terrors, like those of sleepwalking, occur out of stage 3 or stage 4 sleep early during the sleep period (see figure 16). They are associated with tremendous increases of pulse rate, respiratory rate, and blood pressure during the thirty seconds or so it takes to wake up.

Enuresis, the involuntary passage of urine during the night, is most common in children; this condition, too, is found to occur during periods of stage 3 and stage 4 sleep early in the night. It occurs somewhat more frequently in people who have night terrors and/or sleepwalking as well.

All three of these conditions—sleepwalking, night terrors, and enuresis—run in families to a certain extent. They are sometimes called disorders of arousal, since they are not ongoing processes, such as dreams, that would be interrupted by an arousal; rather, the condition is the unusual arousal experience itself.

These three conditions are usually relatively innocuous. They generally do not produce great harm, nor do they often require specific treatment. However, this is not always the case. A man who suffered from severe night terror–sleepwalking episodes caused three

•

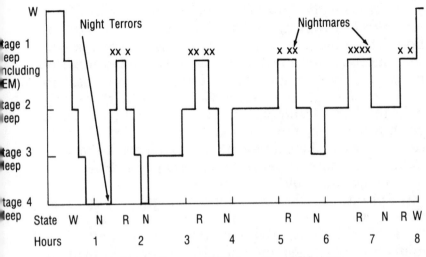

Key: W = wakefulness; N = non-REM sleep; R = REM sleep;
     x = presence and approximate spacing of rapid eye movements

Note: Night terrors occur early (often within an hour of falling asleep), during deep non-REM sleep (stage 4). Nightmares occur toward morning during REM, or dreaming, sleep.

Figure 16. Occurrence of night terrors and nightmares in the sleep laboratory

From *The Nightmare: The Psychology and Biology of Terrifying Dreams* by Dr. Ernest Hartmann. Copyright © 1984 by Ernest Hartmann. Reprinted by permission of the publisher.

deaths during one of these episodes. He had become very tired on a long drive and pulled into a rest area to sleep for a while. About half an hour after falling asleep, he started the car and, according to several observers, seemed to be driving in an erratic fashion with a sort of glazed expression in his eyes. He ended up on the wrong side of a major highway and had a head-on collision in which the deaths occurred. I have seen several other people whose condition was not quite as severe but whose wives or children were hurt by the patient walking and thrashing about in the night during a sleepwalking episode.

Occasionally episodes of night terrors—with and without sleepwalking—occur as a side effect of medication. The antidepressant group of medications is one that can have this effect, but occasionally other medications have been implicated. Certainly if you start to have episodes of terror at night, or if you start walking in your sleep (assuming this is not an old pattern for you), it is worth thinking about whether you have recently started taking a new medication (keep a chart, as outlined in chapter 5). If so, there is a good chance that the medication could be responsible.

Episodes of sleepwalking and night terrors occasionally occur after a cerebrovascular accident, or stroke. Bed-wetting can occur after a stroke or after any injury to the nerves and muscles involved in bladder control; however, this would usually be a problem all day, rather than only in the early night. Finally, someone who has had these conditions, especially sleepwalking and night terrors, throughout life may continue to have them in older age, but the frequency of the episodes usually decreases. Such a person will have become accustomed to the condition and will be happy to see that it is improving. In such a case, the condition is not likely to produce any particular concern or require any particular treatment in older age.

Treatment for these three conditions is usually straightforward. If the condition appears to have been produced by medication, one can stop or change the medication, or one can wait a few weeks, since the sleepwalking or night terrors sometimes occur only once or twice as the body is adjusting to medication. When the condition is produced by a stroke or other central nervous system problem, one needs to treat the stroke or underlying problem; specific treatment for the sleep disorder is not usually required. This holds, too, when sleepwalking or night terrors have been long-term conditions; they do not usually require specific treatment. However, no matter what produces these conditions—especially sleepwalking and night terrors—they are usually aggravated by excessive tired-ness or sleep deprivation; stress, too, can frequently aggravate these problems. Thus, maintaining a regular sleep pattern, avoiding becoming overtired, avoiding alcohol, and avoiding unusually stressful situations (easier said than done!) can be helpful. Counseling and psychotherapy can also be helpful in dealing with stress.

When the situation is serious, safety measures should be instituted. Someone who is prone to sleep-walking or to episodes of sleepwalking that are accom-panied by night terrors should, of course, not sleep near a plate-glass window or near anything else that could cause harm to himself or herself. A night-light should be used in the sleeper's room, and such obsta-cles as extension cords, chairs, and bedroom slippers should be removed from the area around the bed and along any usual walking paths. The sleepwalker should certainly not sleep with a handgun or a knife in a drawer beside the bed.

Medication can reduce or stop the sleepwalking and night terror episodes if they become very serious. Diazepam (Valium) and certain related medications have this effect. However, these drugs can in them-selves produce problems such as confusion and disori-entation in older persons, and since it is often difficult to stop taking them, the "cure" may be more dangerous than the "disease." Diazepam should be taken only in serious situations—in cases where the patient has actu-ally experienced an injury and is continuing to injure himself or herself, by getting up during a sleepwalking episode and walking into a wall or window, for example.

Overall, it is worth keeping in mind that the epi-sodes of night terrors and enuresis and most (but not all) cases of sleepwalking are not in themselves very dangerous. They very seldom become worse, and they are usually more disturbing to others, roommates or spouses, than to the sleeper.

NIGHTMARES

Nightmares, sometimes called dream anxiety attacks, are quite different from night terrors. This difference is confirmed in sleep laboratory studies. Nightmares are long, frightening dreams that wake the sleeper. They are not accompanied by sleepwalking or thrashing about. The sleeper seldom screams out loud, though the nightmares can be very disturbing, and sometimes the sleeper dreams that he or she is screaming. Nightmares, like other dreams, arise out of dreaming (REM) sleep (see figure 16). Nightmares in the laboratory are reported from a long (twenty- to thirty-minute) REM period during the second half of the sleep period—for most people 3:00 A.M. to 7:00 A.M. Unlike night terrors, which have almost no content, the nightmare has a good deal of content. Almost always, it is a long, frightening dream in which the sleeper is in some way vulnerable—being chased, hurt, attacked, or killed.

"I was with a bunch of people at a party when strange lights began to flicker on and off. Someone opened the door, and there were a bunch of thugs out there. They scared me a lot, and I seemed to know some of them. They had sort of a familiar look on their faces. A couple of them started chasing me. I ran away down the street. For a while, it seemed I was paralyzed, and I couldn't get away. I finally ran into a building. One of them came after me and cornered me. He pulled out a knife, and he was just about to stab me when I awoke."

Having a nightmare is frightening but is not necessarily any cause for concern. In fact, at least 50 percent of adults have an occasional nightmare, and nightmares can occur at any age. A study in my laboratory of an extreme group—adults ages twenty to forty who reported nightmares at least once a week (often every night) and reported having them as a lifelong condition—revealed that the participants were in general unusually open people who were creative and had artistic talents but who also appeared vulnerable to certain forms of mental illness. They had "thin boundaries" in many different senses—including being thin-skinned and having a thin, or flexible, sense of group identity and of sexual identity. Although the nightmares sounded terrifying, they were not seen as a major problem by most of the people studied. Some of the artists even made use of their nightmares in their creative work. People in their fifties and sixties who have had nightmares all their lives generally report that as they become older, their nightmares have become less frequent and less frightening but continue to occur.

Nightmares tend to be more frequent and more frightening at times of change and times of stress. Thus, if you have had only an occasional nightmare in the past but have been experiencing considerably more of them recently, it is worth looking into whether there is some source of stress or anxiety that might be responsible. Situations that make you feel helpless or vulnerable may be especially important triggers for nightmares.

Overall, nightmares are seldom a major problem in older persons. However, a sudden appearance of nightmares can be related to medication—usually one of the blood pressure medications known as beta-blockers. In addition to the beta-blockers, several other medications produce or bring out severe nightmares. These are the reserpine group, used in the treatment of high blood pressure and sometimes in the treatment of psychosis, and a group of drugs related to levodopa, used in the treatment of Parkinson's disease.

A nightmare is obviously not contained in a little capsule of medicine. The material for a nightmare must have been lurking inside and have been released or brought out by the medication. We all have in us the material for violent and aggressive fantasies, which can be brought out under the right conditions. One of these conditions is the chemical change that occurs when one takes certain medications.

These nightmares almost always disappear if medication is changed or reduced. Sometimes the medication is essential and cannot be discontinued. In these cases, it is very useful for the patient simply to know that the nightmares can be brought on by the medication and that they do not indicate serious psychological trouble. With this knowledge, people who cannot change their medication may learn simply to live with the nightmares.

BRUXISM

Nocturnal tooth grinding, or bruxism, is a condition like snoring, apnea, or myoclonus that is usually not noticed by the sleeper but is evident to someone else sleeping in the bed or in the same room. It is a fairly common disorder. Bruxism involves grinding the teeth powerfully during the night, making a loud noise—often loud enough to wake up someone else in the room, though the sleeper does not hear the noise. Bruxism can occur at any age. However, it is rare to have it for the first time when you are sixty or seventy. If you have serious bruxism, you may not hear it yourself, but someone who shares your bedroom will notice; or your dentist will notice, since bruxism can cause serious damage to the teeth and gums. Some people have worn down their teeth to mere stubs by nighttime tooth grinding.

Although bruxism is not entirely understood, a few points are well established. First, there is a familial tendency toward bruxism. Thus, if someone in your family is a tooth grinder, you are somewhat more likely than most people to be one too. Bruxism is sometimes caused by slight malformations of the teeth and jaws, so if you have bruxism, it is worth consulting your dentist to see whether you have some malformation that can be corrected. Even if it cannot be corrected, a dentist can make a mouth guard, a sort of rubber or plastic cover for your teeth, that will prevent further tooth damage from bruxism, though it will not prevent the grinding movements themselves.

One factor that makes a difference, at least in some cases of bruxism, is alcohol. Some people develop quite severe bruxism when they have had three or four drinks in the course of an evening, whereas they have no bruxism at all when they do not drink alcohol. Certainly this is not the whole story, but at least in some persons alcohol aggravates bruxism; marijuana or other street drugs seem to have the same effect.

Psychological factors may be important too. Bruxism seems to be more common in people who are somewhat tense or angry. And in just about everyone who has bruxism, it is worse when they are undergoing tense, stressful periods. There is also some indication that bruxism occurs especially in people with suppressed anger—feelings of anger for which one has no adequate outlet. If you grind your teeth a great deal at night, it may be worth exploring this possibility and getting appropriate help.

CARDIOVASCULAR SYMPTOMS

One additional episodic sleep disorder that does occur more commonly in older persons involves cardiovascular symptoms, especially attacks of angina pectoris during sleep. This usually occurs in patients who have the condition during wakefulness as well, but some may have attacks only at night. Angina is a heavy, pressing chest pain produced when the heart muscle receives insufficient oxygen. Angina pain is worth taking seriously whether it occurs at night or in the daytime, since it is sometimes a warning of later, more serious problems such as heart attack. There are many changes in pulse and in blood pressure during periods of REM sleep (see chapter 2), which can temporarily reduce blood flow and oxygen to the heart as well as to other parts of the body; there is one study showing that people with a tendency to attacks of angina have them more often during REM sleep than during any other time.

There are a number of other episodic events classified by the Association of Sleep Disorders Centers (see Appendix A). However, none of them appear to be common in older persons.

◀ 10 ▶

A Diagnostic Guide
to Sleep Problems

This chapter presents a simple guide in tabular form
that starts with your main sleep symptom, or complaint, and comes up with possibilities as to what underlying problem you may have and what to do about
it. For instance, a reader can look in the table first for a
major symptom—"Trouble falling asleep." The reader
then looks in the second column for associated symptoms or related comments—"You drink quite a bit of
coffee, tea, cocoa, colas, or other caffeine-containing
beverages." In the third column the possible problem of
"Caffeine-induced insomnia" is listed, and in the fourth
column a suggestion of what to do—in this case, "Reduce your caffeine intake"—is given.

You may want to find additional information about
your problem elsewhere in this book. Consult the Index
for the appropriate pages.

A DIAGNOSTIC GUIDE TO SLEEP PROBLEMS

If your main symptom is—	And in addition—
Trouble falling asleep (and sometimes remaining asleep)	You have no daytime symptoms, but you mostly sit watching TV, reading, etc.
Trouble falling asleep	You drink quite a bit of coffee, tea, cocoa, colas, or other caffeine-containing beverages.
Trouble falling asleep	You become more alert when you get into bed instead of more sleepy.
Trouble falling asleep	You sleep much better away from home than in your own bed.
Trouble remaining asleep	You have been told that you snore heavily.
Trouble remaining asleep (waking up a lot)	You are very restless and move around a lot in your sleep.
Trouble remaining asleep (waking up a lot)	You are overweight and have increasing blood pressure.
Trouble remaining asleep (waking up a lot)	You have sleep attacks in the daytime, you fall asleep when you don't want to, and you're very tired.

The problem may be—	You should then—
Insufficient activity	Try to increase your mental and/or your physical activity.
Caffeine-induced insomnia	Reduce your caffeine intake.
Psychophysiological insomnia	Use your bed only for sleep. Consider changing beds.
Psychophysiological insomnia	Use your bed only for sleep. Consider changing beds.
Sleep apnea	Seek professional help.
Sleep apnea, nocturnal myoclonus	Seek professional help.
Sleep apnea	Seek professional help.
Sleep apnea, narcolepsy	Seek professional help.

Continued on next page

A DIAGNOSTIC GUIDE TO SLEEP PROBLEMS—*Continued*

If your main symptom is—	And in addition—
Trouble remaining asleep (waking up a lot)	You drink a lot of alcohol in the evening.
Trouble falling asleep and remaining asleep	You recently discontinued or reduced the use of tranquilizers or sleeping pills.
Trouble falling asleep or staying asleep for the past few weeks	Someone close to you has died, or you have experienced some other disturbing event.
Trouble falling asleep and remaining asleep (waking up a lot)	You are sleeping in a different, noisy, or hectic environment.
Falling asleep easily but waking up during the night and/or waking up very early in the morning	You have trouble functioning in the early morning, but you gradually feel better as the day goes on.
Feeling tired and groggy in the morning and unable to function well	You sleep well at night with the help of a sleeping medication.
Trouble falling asleep at your usual bedtime	You have trouble getting up at your usual time, and you're still tired.

The problem may be—	You should then—
Alcohol-related insomnia	Reduce your alcohol consumption. Seek help through counseling, AA, etc.
Rebound insomnia	Wait—give yourself time. (Do not resume or increase the use of sleeping pills or tranquilizers.)
Transient, situational insomnia	Wait. (This is a normal reaction, and nothing specific needs to be done.)
Simple insomnia due to sensitivity and/or sleep disruption	Try to alter your environment by cutting down the noise, light, etc.
Depression	Seek professional help.
Possible buildup effect from too much sleeping medication	Call the physician who prescribed the medication. Make a change.
Jet lag or other rhythm disturbance	If you've just flown from west to east, wait a few days. If not, examine your sleep-wake schedule.

Continued on next page

A DIAGNOSTIC GUIDE TO SLEEP PROBLEMS—*Continued*

If your main symptom is—	And in addition—
Waking up earlier than your usual time	You are tired in the evening and want to go to bed early.
Not feeling tired when you go to bed but often being tired in the daytime	You have a very irregular schedule.
Trouble falling alseep at your regular bedtime but falling asleep all right if you go to bed hours later	The time your body wants to go to sleep keeps getting later and later.
Trouble staying awake until your usual bedtime	You seem to keep getting tired and falling asleep earlier and earlier.
Suddenly falling asleep in the daytime	You feel wonderful, very well rested, after one of these ten- or fifteen-minute attacks.
Suddenly falling asleep in the daytime	You have noticed sudden muscle weakness or sleep paralysis as you wake up or strange hallucinations as you wake up or fall asleep.
Suddenly falling asleep in the daytime	You have been told that you snore heavily and irregularly at night.

The problem may be—	You should then—
Jet lag or other rhythm disturbance	If you've just flown from east to west, wait a few days. If not, examine your sleep-wake schedule.
Irregular sleep-wake pattern	Keep bedtime, waking time, meals, etc., as regular as possible.
Delayed sleep-phase syndrome	Seek professional help.
Advanced sleep-phase syndrome	Seek professional help.
Narcolepsy	Seek professional help.
Narcolepsy	Seek professional help.
Sleep apnea	Seek professional help.

Continued on next page

A DIAGNOSTIC GUIDE TO SLEEP PROBLEMS—*Continued*

If your main symptom is—	And in addition—
Feeling very tired in the daytime and falling asleep when you don't want to	You're not sure whether you snore or have other problems at night.
Feeling tired in the daytime, and it is getting worse over the past year or two	Your blood pressure has been rising.
Feeling tired in the daytime even after your usual amount of sleep	You've been told that you sleep very restlessly— that you kick all the time.
Feeling tired in the daytime even though you get to sleep all right	You have been drinking more alcohol lately (or you are not sure how much you have been drinking lately).
Feeling tired in the daytime	You recently have started a new medication, or your medication has been changed.
Feeling tired in the daytime	You are somewhat overweight, and/or you wake up with headaches, and/or your blood pressure has been rising.
Feeling tired in the daytime	Your muscles often feel strange, as though they have to move—you have "restless legs."

The problem may be—	You should then—
Sleep apnea, nocturnal myoclonus, or any other disorder mentioned in chapter 7	Obtain professional help to determine whether you have a serious condition.
Sleep apnea or a related condition	Seek professional help.
Nocturnal myoclonus	Seek professional help.
Alcohol effects	Discontinue alcohol use. If you find this difficult, obtain help.
Medication effects	Call the physician who prescribed the medication. Make a change.
Sleep apnea	Seek professional help.
Nocturnal myoclonus (associated with restless legs syndrome)	Seek professional help.

Continued on next page

A DIAGNOSTIC GUIDE TO SLEEP PROBLEMS—*Continued*

If your main symptom is—	And in addition—
Waking up in a strange place (not where you went to bed)	Others see you walking at night and have trouble communicating with you.
Screaming at night and striking out, especially an hour or two after you fall asleep	You remember little or nothing, except sometimes waking up scared.
Having long, frightening dreams that wake you up	You do not scream, walk, or strike out.
Complaints from spouse or roommate of a loud grinding sound while you sleep	Occasionally your jaws are sore in the morning.
Your teeth are ground down	Occasionally your jaws are sore in the morning.
Getting lost in the evening and not being able to find your way around the house or yard	You are all right in the morning and afternoon.

The problem may be—	You should then—
Sleepwalking	Avoid overtiredness and alcohol. Consider the possibility of a medication effect. If you are in danger of harming yourself or others, seek professional help.
Night terrors	Avoid overtiredness and alcohol. Consider the possibility of a medication effect. If you are in danger of harming yourself or others, seek professional help.
Nightmares	Usually no treatment is necessary. Consider the possibility of a medication effect.
Bruxism	Check with your dentist.
Bruxism	Check with your dentist.
Sundowning	Leave more lights on. Try to have more people around. Make the evening more like the daytime.

⫷ 11 ⫸

Dreams

Dreaming, of course, is not a sleep disorder; it is an entirely normal part of our lives. However, I think it will be worthwhile for us to spend a few pages considering dreaming for several reasons. First of all, although dreaming is entirely normal, a sudden change in dreaming patterns sometimes causes concern. We will look at what such changes mean and whether they need to be a cause for worry. Secondly, dreaming is an often-neglected part of our mental lives that can sometimes be of positive use to us in self-understanding and overall health.

WHO REMEMBERS DREAMS AND WHEN

We all have three to five dreaming-sleep periods (REM periods) in the course of a night, whether or not we usually remember our dreams. And we are all capable of remembering dreams if we are awakened at the right time. In studies where sleepers have been awakened and asked about dream content, they have almost all reported dreams when awakened from a REM period— especially a long REM period late in the night.

In any particular study, there are always exceptions. Perhaps 10 to 20 percent do not remember a dream or at least do not remember a clear dream from a REM-period awakening. Does this mean some people have no dreams at all? More likely, the nonrecall can be attributed to simple forgetting, fuzziness, repression (an unconscious pushing away of difficult material), or suppression (a conscious decision on the sleeper's part not to mention a dream even though he or she does recall something). The same 10 to 20 percent who could not recall a dream in the study often will remember a dream at other times.

What determines who recalls dreams and who doesn't, or when we recall a dream and when we don't? One factor is simply physiological—the question of how deeply and uninterruptedly we sleep. Those people who sleep extremely well and deeply are less likely to recall dreams than those who sleep less deeply and with more interruptions. This factor makes perfect sense in terms of laboratory studies. We remember dreams primarily when we wake up spontaneously or are awakened by an experimenter during or just after a REM period.

In addition, there are several psychological factors involved. Simply having an interest in dreams produces an increase in dream recall. You, the reader of this book, are somewhat more likely to remember a dream tonight than last night or the night before, simply because you have read a little about dreaming today.

Recall is also related to deeper psychological factors. Those who are interested and fascinated by their own mental lives, who can tolerate ambiguity, and who are intrigued by strange and not very rational mental material in themselves and others are more likely to remember dreams than those who have no interest in fantasy or mental life, or those who are annoyed or frightened by the idea of a lot of strange things going on in their heads.

SUDDEN CHANGES IN DREAMING PATTERNS OR DREAM CONTENT

Generally speaking, most of us have a variety of dreams throughout our lives. Similarly, we recall more or fewer dreams at different times for some of the biological and psychological reasons already noted and for other reasons we don't understand. Simply having more or fewer dreams than usual is not a cause for concern; however, there are a few times when changes in dreaming can signal an important problem. A sudden increase in nightmares, insomnia, and anxiety can sometimes warn one of an impending psychotic episode. In someone who is not particularly anxious or insomniac, the sudden onset of confusing, vivid dreams and/or nightmares may be a result of medication, especially certain medications used for hypertension and for parkinsonism.

There is one other change that may be important. Dreaming changes are sometimes associated with the onset of depression. If you normally dream quite a bit; have a mixture of happy, sad, and frightening dreams; and suddenly find that you are dreaming less (without medication being responsible) and that the few dreams you do have are dark, gloomy, or with few people in them, you may be developing a depressive illness (see pages 75–80). The opposite is true as well. If you are suddenly remembering more dreams and your dreams are becoming more lively and active with more people in them, this may indicate that you have been in a period of depression that is now lifting.

Many people are interested in the question of

whether a sudden, very dramatic dream means any-thing specific: "If I dream that something is burning my stomach, does that mean I am getting an ulcer?" I cannot answer this question based on solid evidence. In most cases there is no actual ulcer or physical problem. There are, however, a number of anecdotal reports suggesting that dreams can sometimes be sensitive to subtle changes in one's body that one is not yet aware of. A man dreams of something squeezing his heart; soon after the dream he begins to have angina attacks and eventually has a heart attack. The most dramatic incident I've heard was of a woman who dreamt that she was lying in the road naked when a motorcycle ran over her breast. She felt a severe pain in her left breast and woke up frightened. She was in psychotherapy and discussed with her therapist for some time the possible psychological meanings of this dream. But a routine breast examination a month after the dream revealed a tumor in her left breast (later successfully removed). Cases of this kind are very rare, but even an occasional occurrence suggests that if you have a really traumatic dream of this kind relating to a specific part of your body, you should at least have a good medical checkup to look into a possible illness.

Another frequent question is, "If I dream that my sister is dying, is she really dying?" This refers to tele-pathic dreams (assuming the sister lives miles away and has been healthy). There has been a lot of serious inter-est in whether telepathy in dreams can actually occur. I have frequently heard of such cases as the following:

"I dreamt my mother [who lives five hundred miles away] was in awful pain and was dying. I woke up, thought about it for a few hours, and then called my father. He told me that my mother had indeed suffered a heart attack that night and was in the hospital."

As a scientist, I would have to say that there is no very solid evidence for telepathy. One careful study, by

Ullman and associates in New York, found positive evidence of telepathy in dreams, but several other studies have failed to confirm this.

It is possible that at least some of the incidents are coincidence or are elaborations after the fact. (Perhaps the dream about the mother had been vague in the daughter's memory, but after she woke up and found that indeed her mother had had an attack, she elaborated and decided, yes, that was exactly what she had dreamt.) Such explanations are not entirely convincing, and there is at least a possibility that there is such a thing as telepathic communication in dreams or elsewhere, though the mechanisms by which this occurs are entirely unknown to us. If I had a vivid dream of this kind, I would certainly call to find out if anything had happened.

MEANINGS AND USES OF DREAMS

All mental activity has a meaning. Our dreams—like our thoughts, waking fantasies, and daydreams—come from our own heads, and they obviously refer to some mixture of recent experiences, memories, wishes, and fears stored in our minds. Does this also mean that dreams can be interpreted? Yes. If you remember many dreams, you will almost certainly have recalled dreams that have some clear relevance to something that was going on in your life.

Some dreams have obvious meanings. A patient starting psychoanalysis often has a dream somewhat like the following (an actual case):

"I was walking along a path in the mountains, and there were dangerous cliffs to one side of me and a kind of yawning pit on the other side. I felt a little bit scared. There was some kind of a large figure, perhaps a man, walking next to me, but I wasn't sure whether he 'was on my side.'"

This dream certainly refers to embarking on the journey of psychoanalysis.

Dreaming involves a part of our minds of which we are not usually aware. There is a great deal in our heads that we are not conscious of at any given time. We walk into a new place or bite into a cookie and are suddenly flooded with old memories and feelings that we thought we had long forgotten. We meet again a member of our family or a friend whom we had pushed out of our lives and "forgotten about," and suddenly we find that far from having forgotten the person, we have simply pushed him or her underground and are still full of feelings, thoughts, and recollections. Dreaming can help us uncover these hidden parts of ourselves.

A man in his fifties dreams, "I was with my brother and some others trying to fix a door. We were trying to fit a key into the lock. I think I finally got it in and opened the door correctly. Suddenly, my mother was there with us. She said something like, 'Well, you are a grown-up man now.' And I said, 'But Mother, you're a seventy-year-old lady.'" This man's mother had died ten years before, and this was the first time he had dreamt about her in some years. The dream led to all kinds of interesting associations about himself, his brother, and his mother—his mother holding the key to mysteries in his life and his brother's life—and thoughts about his relationship with his mother. Did he finally feel grown-up after all these years? This is a problem he struggled with and that perhaps we all struggle with for much of our lives. Are we independent and grown-up, or are we still dependent on our parents? And do we want to be grown-up and "on our own," or do we still cling to patterns of childhood? There are no definitive answers, but our dreams are one way of exploring our own views.

As we become older, we dream to some extent about aging. But we also dream a great deal about youth and childhood. People in their sixties, seventies, and eighties still dream about relationships with their parents, about sexual issues, and about competition with siblings.

"It was a very violent scene . . . some kind of a prison breakout, I think. There were guards and prisoners shooting at each other. The prisoners were trying to get out. I was watching, but somehow I was on the side of the prisoners."

This dream led to all kinds of associations, revealing how the dreamer—a fifty-two-year-old businessman and father of three children—who on the surface appeared to be leading a reasonably peaceful, quiet life, nonetheless had a great deal of angry struggle in him, much of it involving trying to get out from under the influence of his very difficult parents. The dream helped him begin to come to terms with these old feelings.

The dream shows that there are important lifelong issues that we always struggle with in one way or another; perhaps, like the Dutch farmers, we spend our whole lives repairing the dikes. Examining our dreams is a good way of becoming aware of our own dikes and our own repairs.

Even a nightmare or a frightening dream can be interesting and useful. It can sometimes provide a view of how one's mental state is changing. A brilliant woman, a patient in psychoanalysis who had had a difficult childhood and was working on problems in her relationships and her professional life, had many dreams of large, frightening sharks or sharklike monsters coming out of the ocean and chasing or threatening her. These dreams occurred several times before and during psychoanalysis, when she was unsure where her life was headed and when she was reexperiencing childhood fears and childhood helplessness. As she began to understand and overcome some of her fears and her life became more stable, she dreamt several more times of the sharklike monsters, but they looked less threatening and terrifying than before. Finally, at a time when she was finishing treatment and her life and work were going well, she had one final dream of a sharklike monster. It came up out of the water of a swimming pool right next to her, she patted it on the head and rubbed its fur, and it curled up at her feet like a friendly dog!

I'm not discussing here any particular school of dream interpretation. Sometimes associating freely to elements of the dream can lead us in interesting directions. Sometimes the dream itself can be taken as a fascinating total picture. A school of therapists called existentialist would have us simply get into the dream—appreciate the picture, appreciate the feeling, get to know it better, get to know ourselves better: "One time on a mountaintop, there was a strong wind blowing. I was afraid I would be blown over." Here, the existentialist therapist guides the dreamer to a whole series of powerful but half-buried feelings. First, the feeling of being fragile, of being someone who could be blown away, of being in danger. But then, too, the dreamer can become the wind and experience a feeling of power: "I *am* the wind. I am unstoppable. I have immense strength in me. This is kind of fun."

Sometimes a dream can be immediately helpful in bringing about a beneficial change in our lives. We have seen that once in a while a traumatic dream about one's body may signal an illness that we are not yet aware of in our waking lives. More often, however, the dream expresses our wishes, fears, or concerns in dramatic terms. A well-known sleep researcher, a heavy smoker, woke up one morning from a terrible dream. He had dreamt that he had lung cancer; he had seen the X rays indicating extensive involvement of his lungs as well as the lymph nodes. He had realized in the dream that he would die soon and never live to see his children grow up. He woke up in a sad and terrified state. This dream caused him to stop smoking immediately. He did not in fact have lung cancer, but the dream had expressed his concerns more vividly than he could express them in waking life. Since the dream inspired him to stop smoking, it may have been beneficial in preventing lung cancer at some future time.

If you are interested in your dreams even a little bit, it is worth exploring them further. You may think, "It couldn't be an important part of me. I hardly remember any dreams." We all dream; the difference is in how much we remember. You can become more aware of your dreams simply by reading these paragraphs, by paying attention to your dreams, and by deciding you are more interested. And then, if you wish, you can look at your own dreams in different ways, read books about dreams, attend one of the many dream workshops or dream-sharing groups that now exist, or tell a therapist about your dreams and see what you can work out. Exploration of your dreams may lead you to better sleep and a healthier and more satisfying waking life.

◀ 12 ▶

Sleep and Wakefulness— There's More You Can Do

Sleep is an integral part of our overall physical and mental being—and well-being. Even if we do not have a specific sleep problem, our sleep will nonetheless vary a great deal from time to time in quantity, quality, and the satisfaction we get from it. Aspects of our waking life vary as well, and the two are related. Sleep processes and waking processes both change with age. We can learn to understand, accept, and adapt to these changes. We need to get away from the attitude of "Something is wrong—quick, give me a pill to fix it," and get to a gradual understanding of how different aspects of our lives, including sleep and dreaming, interrelate.

SLEEP TIME AND WAKEFULNESS TIME

In one sense, you can think of sleep as an organ, like the heart or the lungs, and as with an organ, it is subject

141

to a number of specific problems or illnesses that can be treated. Obstructive sleep apnea is one of these problems. We can sometimes find precisely what is wrong in the back of the throat and apply corrective measures such as medication, positive airway pressure, or surgery to correct this problem.

But sleep is not just an organ that can have a specific problem. Sleep is a part of being human. Your sleep and your wakefulness together constitute your life, and the quality of one will have a powerful effect on the quality of the other. You organize your sleep-wakefulness pattern; in turn your sleep-wakefulness pattern organizes you. A great deal of your life works circularly. For instance, if you are feeling bad about yourself for one reason or another, you may stop eating regular meals and sleeping at regular times. You may cut your activity level way back—doing things only when you have the energy to do them and not doing anything at all much of the time. Your sleep-wakefulness pattern and your other life patterns become disorganized. Your body hormones and other chemical systems, no longer receiving their usual signals from your activities, lose their regular pattern of changes. Your nervous system picks this up and sends messages to your brain—"Things are disorganized, things are going badly." Your brain should then make some changes. But if you are in the state described, your brain does nothing. The signals coming into your brain saying "Things are in bad shape" simply reinforce your general malaise. You say, "Yeah, that's what I thought. Things are just in bad shape. Everything is going downhill for me. Life is not as much fun as it used to be." Then of course you take even less care of your sleeping and eating. You are even less interested in doing anything in the daytime, and the whole pattern becomes worse.

It can work the other way too. Life is going well. You are really involved in something and are stimulated by your daily activity. You have had some good experiences with someone you love and find that your relationships are strong and satisfying. Now when you wake up, you feel alert. You get meals at regular times. You accomplish a good deal during the day. You feel tired in the evening, go to bed, fall asleep quickly, and sleep well. The next day holds similar promise—you enjoy it. There is sunshine in your life, metaphorically and literally. You get an earlier start. The sun *does* shine on you more, and some recent research suggests that natural sunlight may actually have some antidepressant effect. If so, this effect may add to your good feeling. You feel better. You do more. You feel more tired in the evening. You feel better the next morning. The signals your body receptors send to your brain say, "The world is good. I'm feeling pretty good today." They simply reinforce what your brain has been saying anyway—"Things are going well."

THE SLEEP-WAKEFULNESS RELATIONSHIP

Obviously, awake time and sleep time are related. We only have twenty-four hours each day, and we're always in one state or the other. The more time we spend awake, the less time we have for sleep. But sleep patterns reflect waking patterns. There is a direct relationship between the amount of time one has spent awake and active and the amount of stage 4 sleep—deep, slow-wave sleep—that follows. You recall that stage 4 is thought to be the most physically restorative part of sleep. Studies show that someone who has been awake continuously for sixteen to eighteen hours will have more of this stage 4 sleep than someone who has only been awake eight hours or twelve hours. And there is evidence that persons who are very active—marathon runners, to take an extreme example—have even more stage 4 sleep.

This doesn't mean that one should run a marathon every day, or that no one should ever take a nap. One gets used to one's own body cycles. There are people who do well being very active for six to eight hours, taking a solid afternoon nap, being active for another eight hours, and then getting a night of sleep. In some southern countries, the majority of the population have adopted this pattern. But there is no question that those who spend their days taking short naps, dozing, or doing very little will find it much harder to obtain a good night's sleep afterward.

There are long sleepers, people who always need over nine hours of sleep, and short sleepers, people who always get along on less than six hours. One finding in a study done by myself and associates was that the people who were sure of their purpose and who were busy and involved—sometimes even too busy and involved—were the ones who did not need as much sleep. They slept less, perhaps only five or six hours, but then felt well rested when they got up. They had no sleep problems.

The opposite group, the long sleepers—and there is nothing wrong with being a long sleeper—did not have serious mental problems, but they tended to be "worriers"; their lives were less focused and less intense. They sometimes felt very tired and slept in the daytime; at night, they still needed nine to ten hours of sleep. Their sleep often was not as restful as that of short sleepers. Some of these long sleepers were doing very interesting things; some were making changes in their lives; some were very artistic. But their reorganizing, worrying, and, sometimes, mild depression seemed to lead to the need for more sleep at night. Sleep laboratory studies showed the sleep in this group was long but not as "tightly packed." The long sleepers were not making use of each sleep minute. The short sleepers, who were extremely active, got along fine on five to six hours of sleep, and the studies showed their sleep was "tightly packed." They had a lot of deep, stage 4 sleep early in the night. They seemed to be getting a lot into each minute of sleep; their sleeping state was as intense as their waking state.

In a study done in my laboratory of hundreds of people whose sleep needs varied at different times of their lives, the subjects described their own changing sleep patterns, including times when they were long sleepers and other times when they were short sleepers. When they were asked to describe what was happening in their waking lives at times of reduced sleep need (short, intense sleep), they would describe times when they were intensely involved in something and life was basically going well. Typically, someone who is writing a book or completing a project of some kind would work very hard at this in the daytime, sleep well at night, and find that, in fact, he or she did not require much sleep during these intervals. Intense days are followed by intense sleep, or more solid sleep. When you live a day that is both full of activity and full of meaning, you are then more likely to obtain a solid night's sleep.

WHAT YOU CAN DO

Good, healthy, deep sleep follows good, healthy, active, involved wakefulness. But some of you who perhaps have sleep problems may be saying, "Well, yes, it sounds good, but does it apply to me? What can I do? Some people are just lucky—they just have high energy levels." Some of this energy level probably is constitutional, or built-in. We don't know how much, of course. There is no question that some people are just more energetic, more active, or more involved than others for their entire lives. It is likely that there are genetic factors, though we do not understand them. It is also very likely that factors such as experiences in childhood, early identifications, and whom we adopt as role models play a part. In other words, a person growing up surrounded by active, energetic, happy people is some-what more likely to become that way. This may be in part because of genetics, and it certainly is at least in part a matter of learning and identifying with the grown-ups one lives with.

But, obviously, that is not all. We are given a cer-tain start by our genes. This is added to by our early experiences. But there is a great deal of room for change. I know people—I'm sure we all know people—who were somewhat lethargic, depressed, and un-energetic in their youth, and then something hap-pened. They found themselves. They got interested and got involved and changed in some way. This can happen at any age. Cervantes completed *Don Quixote*, one of the world's masterpieces, at age sixty-eight.

This does not mean that we are all destined to create masterpieces in our later years, but it *can* happen; in less dramatic ways older people are creating every day. It is wise to keep such possibilities in mind.

A person may say, "I don't have any of the serious medical sleep disorders you've discussed. I agree that my poor sleep seems to be related to my waking ac-tivities, but what can I do? I'm just a passive person, I guess. I don't do that much; I don't get involved in things. I just can't get motivated. I just feel empty."

My response would be that "I just feel empty" often means there's conflict. Our minds are filled with forces of many kinds, sometimes in conflict with one another. We all have powerful wishes and powerful feelings ("I love her," "I hate him," "I really want to do _____") conflicting with powerful defenses and prohibi-tions ("You can't do that," "It's not allowed," "That wouldn't be quite fair," "That might be dangerous," "What would people think?" and so on).

In physics when two equal opposing forces meet, there is no movement. When this happens in the mind, one often feels stuck, indecisive, or just "empty." Occa-sionally this is all conscious, and in the open, and then you can examine the different forces and do something.

But most of the time the forces are unconscious; you are not aware of the separate forces or only dimly aware of them. But you are very much aware of the resultant feeling—empty, stuck, unmotivated.

This state of mind is sometimes called inhibition. Closely related to inhibition are certain kinds of depression—not the acute overwhelming depression discussed earlier that is helped by medicine but a more chronic sense of worthlessness, hopelessness, and sometimes guilt. This may be the result of unconscious forces in the mind. There is often a long-standing feeling of anger at a loved person, perhaps a parent or spouse, plus a sense of "I *can't* be angry at him, or her—she's such a devoted mother," "he's such a solid breadwinner," and so on. This sometimes really means "How can I have such ugly feelings? I must be an awful person. It must be all my fault."

Again what often happens is that the original forces—the angry feelings, for instance—are buried, but only the "I'm no good" remains conscious. Since there are many interrelated conflicts of this kind and we all have some of them, most of us feel a little like that at times. Unfortunately, there is no indication that this feeling vanishes as we get older.

It can help to know this. If you can recognize that you are not empty and unmotivated but may instead be inhibited by conflict, you may begin to feel some movement. You can think of your conflicts as something you can dig into and find out about. This digging into oneself is often a worthwhile activity. It can even be creative. It is amazing what you may come up with, and you can seldom know ahead of time.

If you feel down or empty, do something. Get help. If it's an acute situation—a few weeks or months of increasing depression, inability to function, and so on—get medical help, since you may have a serious depression. See a psychiatrist. You may need antidepressant medication. If it's a longer-term situation, you may need help in the form of counseling or psychotherapy. This does not necessarily mean seeing a psychiatrist for years and years. To a certain extent, you can help yourself—through self-analysis or self-therapy. You can use your dreams, your daydreams, and your fantasies to get to know yourself better. Sometimes you can do it with a friend or in a small group of people you feel close to. Sometimes a psychiatrist or another therapist is extremely useful.

Some people stay away from therapy because they feel it is terribly expensive and time-consuming. They feel that the therapist will not be interested in someone past a certain age or that it is not worth pursuing these things at their age. This is not true. Therapists and counselors *are* interested. Growth is possible at any age. Furthermore, the process does not have to be a long, painful, expensive one. It may be worth trying something like the short-term therapy in which you meet with a therapist only ten or twelve times. The limit is set in advance, and it is often surprising how much you uncover and learn about yourself even in that short period. Problems are sometimes resolved even in twelve sessions. If not, you then have a choice of extending the therapy or deciding to try it some other way. There are all kinds of possibilities at any age.

When you bring conflicts to light, understand them, and, if possible, solve them, you may find a lot of energy you never knew was present. At that point you can sit down and write *Don Quixote* or explore your potential in any direction you wish. You can ask, "What have I always wanted to do [to try, to learn] that I haven't had a chance to do? What skills [talents, potentials] do I have that I haven't developed?"

Then you're off and running, developing something inside you that will make you active, possibly physically *and* mentally. If there's something new or creative about it, so much the better. And better sleep will simply be part of a better life.

A

Diagnostic Classification of Sleep Disorders

I. **Disorders of falling asleep and staying asleep (Insomnia)**

  A. Those associated with psychophysiological conditions
    1. Transient and situational occurrences
    2. Persistent conditions

  B. Those associated with psychiatric disorders
    1. Personality disorders
    2. Mood disturbances (e.g., depression)

  C. Those associated with drugs and alcohol
    1. Tolerance to or withdrawal from depressants
    2. Sustained use of stimulants
    3. Sustained use of or withdrawal from other drugs
    4. Chronic alcoholism

  D. Those associated with a sleep-induced respiratory problem
    1. Sleep apnea
    2. Alveolar hypoventilation (reduced oxygen to the lungs)

149

E. Those associated with movement during sleep (muscle jerks)
  1. Nocturnal myoclonus
  2. "Restless legs"

F. Those associated with other medical, toxic, and environmental conditions

G. Those that begin in childhood

H. Other disorders of falling asleep or staying asleep
  1. Repeated REM-sleep interruptions
  2. Atypical features on polysomnograph
  3. Disorders as yet undocumented or undiagnosed

I. Those not considered abnormalities of falling asleep or staying asleep
  1. Short sleeper
  2. Patient complaint with no objective finding by sleep professional
  3. Disorders as yet undocumented or undiagnosed

II. Disorders of excessive sleepiness

A. Those associated with psychophysiological conditions
  1. Transient and situational occurrences
  2. Persistent conditions

B. Those associated with psychiatric disorders
  1. Mood disturbances (e.g., depression)
  2. Other psychiatric disorders not due to an organic disease

C. Those associated with use of drugs or alcohol
  1. Tolerance to or withdrawal from stimulants
  2. Sustained use of depressants

D. Those associated with sleep-induced respiratory problems
  1. Sleep apnea
  2. Alveolar hypoventilation (reduced oxygen to the lungs)

E. Those associated with movement during sleep
   (muscle jerks)
   1. Nocturnal myoclonus
   2. "Restless legs"

F. Narcolepsy

G. Those with no recognizable cause

H. Those associated with other medical, toxic, and
   environmental conditions

I. Other disorders of excessive sleepiness
   1. Intermittent conditions
      a. Klein-Levin syndrome
      b. Menstrual-associated syndrome
   2. Insufficient sleep at night
   3. "Sleep drunkenness"
   4. Disorders as yet undocumented or undiagnosed

J. Those not considered abnormalities of excessive
   sleepiness
   1. Long sleeper
   2. Patient complaint with no objective finding by
      sleep professional

III. Disorders of the sleep-wake schedule

A. Transient conditions
   1. Jet lag
   2. Work-shift change

B. Persistent conditions
   1. Sleeper frequently changing sleep-wake
      schedule
   2. Delayed sleep-phase syndrome
   3. Advanced sleep-phase syndrome
   4. Non-24-hour sleep-wake syndrome
   5. Irregular sleep-wake pattern
   6. Conditions as yet undocumented or
      undiagnosed

IV. Disorders associated with sleep, sleep stages, or partial arousals (episodic events)

A. Sleepwalking

B. Sleep terrors (night terrors)

C. Sleep-related enuresis

D. Others
1. Nightmares
2. Sleep-related epileptic seizures
3. Sleep-related bruxism
4. Sleep-related headbanging
5. Familial sleep paralysis
6. Impaired sleep-related penile tumescence
7. Sleep-related painful erections
8. Sleep-related cluster headaches and chronic severe headaches
9. Sleep-related abnormal swallowing syndrome
10. Sleep-related asthma
11. Sleep-related cardiovascular symptoms
12. Sleep-related gastroesophageal reflux
13. Sleep-related blood changes
14. Asymptomatic polysomnographic finding
15. Disorders as yet undocumented or undiagnosed

B

Directory of Sleep Disorders Centers

Alabama

Sleep Disorders Center of
Alabama
Baptist Medical Center
Montclair
800 Montclair Road
Birmingham, AL 35213
205-592-5650

Sleep/Wake Disorders
Center
University of Alabama
University Station
Birmingham, AL 35294
205-934-7110

Sleep Disorders Center
Children's Hospital of
Alabama
1600 7th Avenue South
Birmingham, AL 35233
205-939-9386

*Sleep Disorders Laboratory
Carraway Methodist
Medical Center
1600 26th Street North
Birmingham, AL 35234
205-226-6164

*Sleep Disorders
Center
Southeast Alabama
Medical Center
PO Drawer 6987
Dothan, AL 36302
205-793-8134

*North Alabama Sleep
Disorders Center
Huntsville Hospital
101 Sivley Road
Huntsville, AL 35801
205-533-8020

* Provisional member as of January 1, 1987

153

*Knollwood Sleep Disorders
Center
Knollwood Long Term
Care Hospital
PO Box 9813
Mobile, AL 36691
205-666-7700

*Sleep Disorders Center
Mobile Infirmary Medical
Center
PO Box 2144
Mobile, AL 36652
205-431-2400

Sleep Disorders Diagnostic
& Research Center
University of Arkansas for
Medical Sciences
4301 W. Markham, Slot
555
Little Rock, AR 72205
501-661-5528

*Sleep Disorders Center
St. Vincent Infirmary
No. 2 St. Vincent Circle
Little Rock, AR 72205
501-660-3011

Arizona

Sleep Disorders Center
Good Samaritan Medical
Center
1111 E. McDowell Road
Phoenix, AZ 85006
602-239-5815

Sleep Disorders Center
University of Arizona
1501 N. Campbell Avenue
Tucson, AZ 85724
602-626-6112

Arkansas

*Sleep Disorders Center
Baptist Medical Center
9601 I-630, Exit 7
Little Rock, AR 72205
501-227-4750

California

WMCA Sleep Disorders
Center
Western Medical
Center–Anaheim
1025 S. Anaheim Boulevard
Anaheim, CA 92805
714-491-1159

*Sleep Disorders Center
Downey Community
Hospital
11500 Brookshire Avenue
Downey, CA 90241
213-806-5280

*Sleep Disorders Institute
St. Jude Hospital and
Rehabilitation Center
101 E. Valencia Mesa Drive
Fullerton, CA 92634
714-871-3280

Sleep Disorders Center
Scripps Clinic and Research
    Foundation
10666 N. Torrey Pines Road
La Jolla, CA 92037
619-455-8087

*Sleep Disorders Center
Grossmont District Hospital
PO Box 158
La Mesa, CA 92044
619-465-0711

*Loma Linda Sleep
    Disorders Center
Veterans Administration
    Hospital
11201 Benton Street
Loma Linda, CA 92354
714-825-7084

UCLA Sleep Disorders
    Clinic
Department of Neurology
710 Westwood Plaza
Room 1184 RNRC
Los Angeles, CA 90024
213-206-8005

*Sleep Disorders Center
Hospital of the Good
    Samaritan
616 S. Witmer Street
Los Angeles, CA 90017
213-977-2206

Sleep Disorders Center
Holy Cross Hospital
15031 Rinaldi Street
Mission Hills, CA 91345
818-898-4639

*Sleep Disorders Center
Hoag Memorial Hospital
    Presbyterian
301 Newport Boulevard
Newport Beach, CA 92663
714-760-5505

Sleep Disorders Center
University of California
    Irvine Medical Center
101 City Drive South
Orange, CA 92668
714-634-5777

*Sleep Disorders Center
Pomona Valley
    Community Hospital
1798 N. Garey Avenue
Pomona, CA 91767
714-623-8715

Sleep Disorders Center
Sequoia Hospital
Whipple and Alameda
    Streets
Redwood City, CA 94062
415-367-5620

San Diego Regional Sleep
    Disorders Center
Harbor View Medical
    Center & Hospital
120 Elm Street
San Diego, CA 92101
619-232-0537

Sleep Disorders Clinic &
    Research Center
St. Mary's Hospital
450 Stanyan Street
San Francisco, CA 94117
415-750-5579

*Sleep Disorders Center
Pacific Presbyterian Medical
  Center
PO Box 7999
San Francisco, CA 94120
415-923-3336

*Sleep Disorders Center
San Jose Hospital
675 E. Santa Clara Street
San Jose, CA 95112
408-977-4445

*Sleep Disorders Center
South Coast Medical Center
31872 Coast Highway
South Laguna, CA 92677
714-499-1311

Sleep Disorders Program
Stanford University Medical
  Center
Hoover Pavilion-2nd Floor
Stanford, CA 94305
415-723-6601

Sleep Disorders Center
Torrance Memorial Hospital
3330 Lomita Boulevard
Torrance, CA 90509
213-235-9110

Colorado

Sleep Disorders Center
Presbyterian Medical Center
1719 E. 19th Avenue
Denver, CO 80218
303-839-6447

Sleep Disorders Center
University of Colorado Health
  Sciences Center
700 Delaware Street
Denver, CO 80204
303-592-7278

*Porter Regional Sleep Disorders
  Center
Porter Memorial Hospital
2525 S. Downing Street
Denver, CO 80210
303-744-6561

Connecticut

Sleep Disorders Center
Griffin Hospital
130 Division Street
Derby, CT 06418
203-735-7421

*Sleep Disorders Center
Mount Sinai Hospital
500 Blue Hills Avenue
Hartford, CT 06112
203-242-4431

New Haven Sleep Disorders
  Center
100 York Street
University Towers
New Haven, CT 06511
203-776-9578

District of Columbia

*Sleep Disorders Center
Georgetown University
  Hospital
3800 Reservoir Road, NW
Washington, DC 20007
202-625-2697

Florida

Sleep Disorders Center
Mt. Sinai Medical Center
4300 Alton Road
Miami Beach, FL 33140
305-674-2613

*Sleep Disorders Center
Tallahassee Memorial
   Regional Medical Center
Magnolia Drive &
   Miccosukee Road
Tallahassee, FL 32308
904-681-1155

*Sleep Disorders Center
Good Samaritan Hospital
PO Box 3166
West Palm Beach, FL 33402
305-655-5511

Georgia

Sleep Disorders Center
Northside Hospital
1000 Johnson Ferry Road
Atlanta, GA 30342
404-851-8135

*Sleep Disorders Center
Memorial Medical Center,
   Inc.
PO Box 23089
Savannah, GA 31403
912-356-8326

Hawaii

Sleep Disorders Center
Straub Clinic and Hospital
888 South King Street
Honolulu, HI 96813
808-523-2311

Idaho

*Idaho Sleep Disorders
   Center
St. Luke's Regional
   Medical Center
190 E. Bannock Street
Boise, ID 83712
208-386-2440

Illinois

Sleep Disorders Center
University of Chicago
5841 S. Maryland Avenue
PO Box 425
Chicago, IL 60637
312-962-1780

Sleep Disorders Center
Rush–Presbyterian–St.
   Luke's Hospital
1753 W. Congress Parkway
Chicago, IL 60612
312-942-5440

*Sleep Disorders Center
Evanston Hospital
2650 Ridge Avenue
Evanston, IL 60201
312-492-4983

*Sleep Disorders Center
Neurology Service
Veterans Hospital
Hines, IL 60141
312-343-7200

Sleep Disorders Center
Methodist Medical Center
   of Illinois
221 N.E. Glen Oak Avenue
Peoria, IL 61636
309-672-4966

*Sleep Disorders Clinic and
   Laboratory
Carle Foundation Hospital
611 W. Park Street
Urbana, IL 61801
217-337-3364

Indiana

*Sleep Disorders Center
St. Mary's Medical Center
3700 Washington Avenue
Evansville, IN 47750
812-479-4257

*Regional Sleep Studies
   Laboratory
Lutheran Hospital of Fort
   Wayne, Inc.
3024 Fairfield Avenue
Fort Wayne, IN 46807
219-458-2001

Sleep Disorders Center
Winona Memorial Hospital
3232 N. Meridian Street
Indianapolis, IN 46208
317-927-2100

*Sleep Disorders Laboratory
St. Vincent Hospital
2001 W. 86th Street
Indianapolis, IN 46260
317-871-2152

*Sleep/Wake Disorders
   Center
Community Hospital of
   Indiana
1500 N. Ritter Avenue
Indianapolis, IN 46219
317-353-4275

*Sleep Disorders Diagnostic
   Center
Methodist Hospital of
   Indiana
1801 N. Senate Boulevard
Indianapolis, IN 46202
317-929-5710

*Sleep Disorders Center
Lafayette Home Hospital
2400 South Street
Lafayette, IN 47903
317-447-6811

Iowa

*Sleep Disorders Center
St. Luke's Hospital
1227 E. Rusholme Street
Davenport, IA 52803
319-326-6740

*Sleep Disorders Center
Iowa Methodist Medical
   Center
1200 Pleasant Street
Des Moines, IA 50308
515-283-6207

*Sleep Disorders Center
Department of Neurology
University of Iowa
   Hospitals and Clinics
Iowa City, IA 52242
319-356-2571

Kansas

*Sleep Disorders Center
Wesley Medical Center
550 N. Hillside Street
Wichita, KS 67214
316-688-2660

Kentucky

*Sleep Disorders Center
St. Joseph's Hospital
1 St. Joseph Drive
Lexington, KY 40504
606-278-3436

Sleep Disorders Center
Humana Hospital
  Audubon
One Audubon Plaza Drive
Louisville, KY 40217
502-636-7459

Louisiana

Tulane Sleep Disorders
  Center
Department of Psychiatry
  and Neurology
1415 Tulane Avenue
New Orleans, LA 70112
504-587-7457

*Sleep Disorders Center
Willis-Knighton Medical
  Center
2600 Greenwood Road
Shreveport, LA 71103
318-632-4823

Maryland

Sleep Disorders Center
Francis Scott Key Medical
  Center
Johns Hopkins University
Baltimore, MD 21224
301-955-0571

*Maryland Sleep Diagnostic
  Center
8415 Bellona Avenue
Ruxton Towers, Suite 211
Baltimore, MD 21204
301-494-9773

National Capital Sleep
  Center
4520 E. West Highway
#406
Bethesda, MD 20814
301-656-9515

Massachusetts

*Sleep Disorders Center
Boston University Medical
  Center
75 E. Newton Street
Boston, MA 02146
617-247-5206

*Sleep Disorders Center
Boston Children's Hospital
300 Longwood Avenue
Boston, MA 02115
617-735-6242

*Sleep Disorders Unit
Beth Israel Hospital
330 Brookline Avenue
Boston, MA 02215
617-735-3237

*Sleep-Wake Disorders Unit
University of
  Massachusetts
55 Lake Avenue North
Worcester, MA 01605
617-856-3802

Michigan

*Sleep/Wake Disorders Unit
Veterans Administration
    Medical Center
Southfield Road & Outer
    Drive
Allen Park, MI 48101
313-562-6000

*Sleep Disorders Clinic
Catherine McAuley Health
    Center
PO Box 995
Ann Arbor, MI 48106
313-572-3093

*Sleep Disorders Center
Taubman Center 1920/0316
1500 E. Medical Center
    Drive
Ann Arbor, MI 48109
313-936-9068

Sleep Disorders Center
Henry Ford Hospital
2799 W. Grand Boulevard
Detroit, MI 48202
313-972-1800

*Sleep Disorders Center
Butterworth Hospital
100 Michigan Street, NE
Grand Rapids, MI 49503
616-774-1695

Sleep Disorders Center
Ingham Medical Center
401 W. Greenlawn Avenue
Lansing, MI 48909
517-374-2510

*Sleep Disorders Center
Traverse City Osteopathic
    Hospital
550 Munson Avenue
Traverse City, MI 49684
616-922-8600

*Bloomfield Institute for
    Sleep
Beaumont Hospital
    Medical Building
44199 Dequindre Road
Suite 403
Troy, MI 48098
313-879-0707

Minnesota

*Duluth Regional Sleep
    Disorders Center
St. Mary's Medical Center
407 E. Third Street
Duluth, MN 55805
218-726-4543

*Sleep Disorders Center
Fairview Southdale
    Hospital
6401 France Avenue South
Edina, MN 55435
612-924-5058

Sleep Disorders Center
Neurology Department
Hennepin County Medical
    Center
Minneapolis, MN 55415
612-347-6288

*Sleep Disorders Center
Abbott Northwestern
   Hospital
800 E. 28th Street at
   Chicago Avenue
Minneapolis, MN 55407
612-874-4257

Sleep Disorders Center
Mayo Clinic
200 1st Street, SW
Rochester, MN 55905
507-286-8900

Sleep Disorders Center
Methodist Hospital
6500 Excelsior Boulevard
St. Louis Park, MN 55426
612-932-6083

*Sleep Diagnostic Center
St. Joseph's Hospital
69 W. Exchange Street
St. Paul, MN 55102
612-291-3682

Mississippi

*Gulf Coast Center for
   Sleep Disorders
Gulf Coast Community
   Hospital
4642 W. Beach Boulevard
Biloxi, MS 39531
601-388-6711

*Sleep Disorders Center
Memorial Hospital at
   Gulfport
PO Box 1810
Gulfport, MS 39501
601-865-3489

*Sleep Disorders Center
Forrest General Hospital
PO Box 16389
Hattiesburg, MS 39401
601-264-4219

Sleep Disorders Center
Division of Somnology
University of Mississippi
Jackson, MS 39216
601-987-5552

Missouri

Sleep Disorders Center
Research Medical Center
2316 E. Meyer Boulevard
Kansas City, MO 64132
816-276-4222

*Sleep Disorders Center
St. Mary's Hospital
28th & Main Streets
Kansas City, MO 64108
816-756-2651

Sleep Disorders Center
St. Louis University
   Medical Center
1221 S. Grand Boulevard
St. Louis, MO 63104
314-577-8705

Sleep Disorders Center
Deaconess Hospital
6150 Oakland Avenue
St. Louis, MO 63139
314-768-3100

*Sleep Disorders Center
L.E. Cox Medical Center
3801 S. National Avenue
Springfield, MO 65807
417-885-6189

Nebraska

*Sleep Physiology Center
Lincoln General Hospital
2300 S. 16th Street
Lincoln, NE 68502
402-473-5338

*Sleep Disorders Center
Lutheran Medical Center
515 S. 26th Street
Omaha, NE 68103
402-536-6352

New Hampshire

*Sleep-Wake Disorders
  Center
Hampstead Hospital
East Road
Hampstead, NH 03841
603-329-5311

Dartmouth-Hitchcock
  Sleep Disorders Center
Department of Psychiatry
Dartmouth Medical School
Hanover, NH 03756
603-646-7534

New York

Sleep-Wake Disorders
  Center
Montefiore Hospital
111 E. 210th Street
Bronx, NY 10467
212-920-4841

*Sleep Disorders Center of
  Western New York
Millard Fillmore Hospital
3 Gates Circle
Buffalo, NY 14209
716-884-9253

*Sleep Disorders Center
Winthrop–University
  Hospital
259 1st Street
Mineola, NY 11501
516-663-2005

Sleep Disorders Center
Columbia Presbyterian
  Medical Center
161 Fort Washington
  Avenue
New York, NY 10032
212-305-1860

Sleep Disorders Center
St. Mary's Hospital
89 Genesee Street
Rochester, NY 14611
716-464-3391

Sleep Disorders Center
Department of Psychiatry
State University of New
  York at Stony Brook
Stony Brook, NY 11794
516-444-2916

Sleep-Wake Disorders Center
New York Hospital–Cornell
  Medical Center
21 Bloomingdale Road
White Plains, NY 10605
914-997-5751

North Carolina

*Sleep Disorders Center
Charlotte Memorial
  Hospital
PO Box 32861
Charlotte, NC 28232
704-338-2121

*Sleep Disorders Center
Duke University Medical
  Center
PO Box 2905
Durham, NC 27710
919-681-3344

*Sleep Disorders Center
Moses H. Cone Memorial
  Hospital
1200 N. Elm Street
Greensboro, NC 27401
919-379-4406

North Dakota

Sleep Disorders Center
St. Luke's Hospital
5th Street at Mills Avenue
Fargo, ND 58122
701-280-5673

Ohio

Sleep Disorders Center
Mercy Hospital of Fairfield
1275 E. Kemper Road
Cincinnati, OH 45246
513-671-3101

Sleep Disorders Center
Bethesda Oak Hospital
619 Oak Street
Cincinnati, OH 45206
513-569-6320

Sleep Disorders Center
Department of Neurology
Cleveland Clinic
9500 Euclid Avenue
Cleveland, OH 44106
216-444-8732

Sleep Disorders Evaluation
  Center
Ohio State University
  Medical Center
473 W. 12th Avenue
Columbus, OH 43210
614-421-8296

Sleep/Wake Disorders
  Center
Miami Valley Hospital
30 Apple Street
Suite G200
Dayton, OH 45409
513-220-2515

*Sleep Disorders Center
Southview Hospital
1997 Miamisburg-
  Centerville Road
Dayton, OH 45459
513-439-6265

*Northwest Ohio Sleep
   Disorders Center
Toledo Hospital
2142 N. Cove Boulevard
Toledo, OH 43606
419-471-5629

Oklahoma

Sleep Disorders Center
Presbyterian Hospital
N.E. 13th at Lincoln
   Boulevard
Oklahoma City, OK 73104
405-271-6312

Oregon

Sleep Disorders Program
Good Samaritan Hospital
2222 N.W. Lovejoy Street
Portland, OR 97210
503-229-8311

Pennsylvania

Sleep Disorders Center
Jefferson Medical College
1015 Walnut Street, Third
   Floor
Philadelphia, PA 19107
215-928-6175

Sleep Disorders Center
Medical College of
   Pennsylvania
3300 Henry Avenue
Philadelphia, PA 19129
215-842-4250

*Sleep Disorders Center
Hospital of the University
   of Pennsylvania
3400 Spruce Street
11 Gates
Philadelphia, PA 19104
215-662-2833

Sleep Disorders Center
Western Psychiatric
   Institute
3811 O'Hara Street
Pittsburgh, PA 15213
412-624-2246

Sleep Disorders Center
Department of Neurology
Crozer-Chester Medical
   Center
Upland-Chester, PA 19013
215-447-2689

South Carolina

*Sleep Disorders Center
Baptist Medical Center
Taylor at Marion Streets
Columbia, SC 29220
803-771-5557

*Sleep Disorders Center
Spartanburg Regional
   Medical Center
101 E. Wood Street
Spartanburg, SC 29303
803-591-6524

South Dakota

*Rushmore Diagnostic
Center for Sleep
Disorders
Rushmore National Health
Systems
353 Fairmont Boulevard
PO Box 6000
Rapid City, SD 57709
605-341-8010

*Sleep Disorders Center
Sioux Valley Hospital
1100 S. Euclid Avenue
Sioux Falls, SD 57117
605-333-6302

Tennessee

Sleep Disorders Center
St. Mary's Medical Center
Oak Hill Avenue
Knoxville, TN 37917
615-971-6011

*Sleep Disorders Center
Ft. Sanders Regional
Medical Center
1901 W. Clinch Avenue
Knoxville, TN 37916
615-971-1375

Sleep Disorders Center
Baptist Memorial Hospital
899 Madison Avenue
Memphis, TN 38146
901-522-5704

Sleep Disorders Center
Saint Thomas Hospital
PO Box 380
Nashville, TN 37202
615-386-2068

Texas

Sleep-Wake Disorders
Center
Presbyterian Hospital
8200 Walnut Hill Lane
Dallas, TX 75231
214-696-8563

Sleep Disorders Center
Sun Towers Hospital
1801 N. Oregon Street
El Paso, TX 79902
915-532-6281

Sleep Disorders Center
All Saints Episcopal
Hospital
1400 8th Avenue
Fort Worth, TX 76104
817-927-6120

*Sleep Disorders Center
Sam Houston Memorial
Hospital
8300 Waterbury Drive
Suite 350
Houston, TX 77055
713-973-6483

Sleep Disorders Center
Department of Psychiatry
Baylor College of Medicine
Houston, TX 77030
713-799-4886

*Center for Sleep Disorders
Lubbock General Hospital
PO Box 5980
Lubbock, TX 79417
806-743-2020

*West Texas Regional Sleep
  Disorders Center
Odessa Women's and
  Children's Hospital
PO Box 4859
Odessa, TX 79760
915-334-8352

*Sleep Disorders Center
Pasadena Bayshore
  Medical Center
4000 Spencer Highway
Pasadena, TX 71504
713-944-6666

*Center for Sleep Disorders
  Medicine
Department of Psychiatry
University of Texas Health
  Science Center
7703 Floyd Curl Drive
San Antonio, TX 78284
512-691-7531

Humana Sleep Disorders
  Center
1303 McCullough Avenue
Suite 447
San Antonio, TX 78212
512-223-4057

Sleep Disorders Center
Scott and White Clinic
2401 S. 31st Street
Temple, TX 76508
817-774-2554

Utah

*Sleep Disorders Center
Utah Neurological Clinic
1055 N. 300 West
Suite 400
Provo, UT 84604
801-379-7400

Intermountain Sleep
  Disorders Center
Latter Day Saints Hospital
325 8th Avenue
Salt Lake City, UT 84143
801-321-3417

Virginia

Sleep Disorders Center
Norfolk General Hospital
600 Gresham Drive
Norfolk, VA 23507
804-628-3322

*Sleep Disorders Center
Chippenham Hospital
7101 Jahnke Road
Richmond, VA 23225
804-320-3911

*Sleep Disorders Center
Community Hospital of
  Roanoke Valley
PO Box 12946
Roanoke, VA 24029
703-985-8435

Washington

Sleep Disorders Center
Providence Medical Center
500 17th Avenue, C-34008
Seattle, WA 98124
206-326-5366

West Virginia

*Sleep Disorders Center
Charleston Area Medical
Center
PO Box 1393
Charleston, WV 25325
304-348-7507

Wisconsin

Sleep Disorders Center
Gundersen Clinic, Ltd.
1836 South Avenue
La Crosse, WI 54601
608-782-7300

*Sleep Disorders Center
University Hospital &
Clinics
600 Highland Avenue
Madison, WI 53792
608-263-7050

*Milwaukee Regional Sleep
Disorders Center
Columbia Hospital
2025 E. Newport Avenue
Milwaukee, WI 53211
414-961-4650

*Sleep Disorders Center
Children's Hospital of
Wisconsin
1700 W. Wisconsin Avenue
PO Box 1997
Milwaukee, WI 53201
414-931-4016

*Sleep/Wake Disorders
Center
St. Mary's Hospital
2323 N. Lake Drive
Milwaukee, WI 53201
414-225-8032

For further information, contact

The Association for Professional Sleep Societies
609 Second Street, SW
Rochester, MN 55902

There are a number of excellent sleep disorders centers
that may not appear on this list. For further information
about them, call the department of psychiatry or
neurology at a medical school or hospital in your area.

C

Directory of Sleep Disorders Specialists

Alabama

Vernon Pegram, Ph.D.
Sleep Disorders Center
Baptist Medical Center
  Montclair
800 Montclair Road
Birmingham, AL 35213
205-592-5650

Virgil Wooten, M.D.
Sleep/Wake Disorders
  Center
University of Alabama
University Station
Birmingham, AL 35294
205-934-4107

Alaska

Carla Hellekson, M.D.
University of Alaska
1919 Lathrop
Drawer 30
Fairbanks, AK 99701
907-452-1739

Arizona

Colin R. Bamford, M.D.
Department of Neurology
University of Arizona
  College of Medicine
1601 Campbell Avenue
Tucson, AZ 85724
602-626-6568

Richard M. Riedy, M.D.
1130 E. McDowell Road
Suite B-7
Phoenix, AZ 85006
602-258-4951

California

Sonia Ancoli-Israel, Ph.D.
Sleep Disorders Clinic
116A Veterans
    Administration Medical
    Center
3350 La Jolla Village Drive
San Diego, CA 92161
619-453-7500

Donna Arand, Ph.D.
UCLA Sleep Disorders
    Clinic
710 Westwood Plaza
Los Angeles, CA 90024
213-206-8005

Roger J. Balogh, M.D.
3158 Altamonte Drive
Beale AFB, CA 95903
916-634-2248

Donald Bliwise, Ph.D.
Sleep Disorders Center
Stanford University Medical
    School
Stanford, CA 94305
415-497-6601

Michael H. Bonnet, Ph.D.
2219 Bentley Avenue, #301
Los Angeles, CA 90064
714-825-7084

Richard M. Coleman, Ph.D.
473 Live Oak Drive
Mill Valley, CA 94941
415-497-6601

William C. Dement, M.D.,
    Ph.D.
440 Gerona Road
Stanford, CA 94305
415-723-6606

Christian Guilleminault,
    M.D.
Sleep Disorders Center
Stanford Medical Center
TD 114
Stanford, CA 94305
415-723-8131

Lawrence W. Kneisley,
    M.D.
3440 W. Lomita Boulevard
#327
Torrance, CA 90505
213-530-8822

Dennis McGinty, Ph.D.
Veterans Administration
    Hospital
16111 Plummer Street
Sepulveda, CA 91343
213-891-2403

Stuart J. Menn, M.D.
Sleep Disorders Center
Scripps Clinic
10666 N. Torrey Pines Road
La Jolla, CA 92037
619-455-8087

Laughton Miles, M.D.
801 Welch Road, Suite 209
Palo Alto, CA 94304
415-326-1462

Merrill M. Mitler, Ph.D.
Sleep Disorders Center
Scripps Clinic
10666 N. Torrey Pines Road
La Jolla, CA 92037
619-455-8087

Sarah S. Mosko, Ph.D.
Department of Neurology
University of California
   Irvine Medical Center
101 City Drive South
Orange, CA 92668
714-634-5778

Elliott R. Phillips, M.D.
Sleep Disorders Center
15031 Rinaldi Street
Mission Hills, CA 91345
818-898-4639

Jon F. Sassin, M.D.
101 The City Drive, South
Orange, CA 92668
714-634-5777

Renata Shaforenko, M.D.
Sleep Disorders Center
Scripps Clinic
10666 N. Torrey Pines Road
La Jolla, CA 92037
619-455-8087

Cheryl L. Spinweber, Ph.D.
Behavioral
   Psychopharmacology
Naval Hospital
Building 36-4
San Diego, CA 92134
619-233-2481

Michael McClain Stevenson,
   Ph.D.
Sleep Disorders Center
Holy Cross Hospital
15031 Rinaldi Street
Mission Hills, CA 91345
818-898-4639

Joel B. Younger, M.D.
10532 Wulff Drive
Villa Park, CA 92667
714-739-1125

Colorado

Eric Hoddes, Ph.D.
1801 Williams Street
Suite 300
Denver, CO 80218
303-355-8800

Martin Reite, M.D.
4200 E. 9th Avenue
PO Box C268
Denver, CO 80262
303-394-7743

John Zimmerman, Ph.D.
700 Delaware Street
Davis Pavilion
Denver, CO 80204
303-394-8887

Connecticut

Deborah E. Sewitch, Ph.D.
Sleep Disorders Center
Griffin Hospital
130 Division Street
Derby, CT 06418
203-735-7421

Robert Watson, Ph.D.
Sleep Disorders Center
Griffin Hospital
130 Division Street
Derby, CT 06418
203-735-7421

Florida

Martin A. Cohn, M.D.
Sleep Disorders Center
Mt. Sinai Medical Center
4300 Alton Road
Miami Beach, FL 33140
305-674-2610

Lawrence Scrima, Ph.D.
Sleep Evaluation Center
University of Miami
  Medical School
Miami, FL 33136
305-547-5926

Illinois

Rosalind Cartwright, Ph.D.
Psychology and Social
  Services
Rush–Presbyterian–
  St. Luke's Hospital
1753 W. Congress Parkway
Chicago, IL 60612
312-942-5000

Robert A. Gross, M.D.
251 E. Chicago Avenue
#930
Chicago, IL 60611
312-266-2389

Howard M. Kravitz, D.O.
8722 N. Springfield Avenue
Skokie, IL 60076
312-942-5440

Henry W. Lahmeyer, M.D.
Department of Psychiatry
University of Illinois
912 S. Wood Street
513A NPI
Chicago, IL 60612
312-996-5266

C. Duane Morgan, M.D.
2907 Winterberry Lane
Peoria, IL 61604
309-686-9214

Richard Rosenberg, Ph.D.
Division of Neurology
Evanston Hospital
2650 Ridge Avenue
Evanston, IL 60201
312-492-2000

Jean-Paul Spire, M.D.
University of Chicago
5841 S. Maryland Avenue
PO Box 425
Chicago, IL 60637
312-962-1782

Kentucky

Carl P. Browman, Ph.D.
Humana Hospital Audubon
One Audubon Plaze Drive
Louisville, KY 40217
502-636-7459

Robert Granacher, M.D.
St. Joseph Office Park
1401 Harrodsburg Road
Lexington, KY 40504
606-278-0317

Maryland

Richard P. Allen, Ph.D.
Johns Hopkins Sleep
  Disorders Center
4940 Eastern Avenue
Baltimore, MD 21224
301-955-0571

David Buchholz, M.D.
Johns Hopkins Hospital
600 N. Wolfe Street
Meyer 1-130
Baltimore, MD 21205
301-955-5348

Ronald P. Lesser, M.D.
Johns Hopkins Hospital
600 N. Wolfe Street
Meyer 2-147
Baltimore, MD 21205
301-955-6540

Wallace Mendelson, M.D.
National Capital Sleep
  Disorders Center
4520 E. West Highway
Suite 406
Bethesda, MD 20814
301-496-2141

Massachusetts

Michael P. Biber, M.D.
1269 Beacon Street
Brookline, MA 02146
617-277-5050

Charles A. Czeisler, M.D.
Neuroendocrinology
  Laboratory
Brigham & Women's
  Hospital
221 Longwood Avenue
Room 505
Boston, MA 02115
617-732-4011

Richard Ferber, M.D.
Center for Pediatric Sleep
  Disorders
Children's Hospital
300 Longwood Avenue
Boston, MA 02115
617-735-6663

Ernest Hartmann, M.D.
170 Morton Street
Boston, MA 02130
617-243-6624

Sandra Horowitz, M.D.
14 Dartmouth Drive
Framingham, MA 01701
617-877-7287

George F. Howard III, M.D.
Boston University Medical
  Center
75 E. Newton Street
Boston, MA 02115
617-247-5203

Michigan

Sheldon Kapen, M.D.
Department of Neurology
Veterans Administration
  Medical Center
Southfield and Outer Drive
Allen Park, MI 48101
313-562-6000

Timothy Roehrs, Ph.D.
Sleep Disorders Center
Henry Ford Hospital
2921 W. Grand Boulevard
Detroit, MI 48202
313-972-1800

Thomas Roth, Ph.D.
Sleep Disorders Center
Henry Ford Hospital
2921 W. Grand Boulevard
Detroit, MI 48202
313-972-1800

Rahul Sangal, M.D.
Bloomfield Institute for
  Sleep Related Disorders
853 Woodward
Pontiac, MI 48053
313-338-6200

James E. Shipley, M.D.
Sleep/Depression Unit
1500 E. Medical Center
  Drive
UH-D9702-0118
Ann Arbor, MI 48109
313-936-4401

Robert C. Smith, M.D.
Department of Medicine
Michigan State University
B301 Clinical Center
East Lansing, MI 48824
517-355-6516

Kenneth E. Starz, M.D.
Upjohn Company
7000 Portage Road
Kalamazoo, MI 49001
616-323-6300

Robert M. Wittig, M.D.
Sleep Disorders Center
Henry Ford Hospital
2921 W. Grand Boulevard
Detroit, MI 48202
313-972-1800

Frank Zorick, M.D.
Sleep Disorders Center
Henry Ford Hospital
2921 W. Grand Boulevard
Detroit, MI 48202
313-972-1800

Minnesota

Paul Fredrickson, M.D.
Sleep Disorders Center
Mayo Clinic
200 S.W. 1st Street
Rochester, MN 55905
507-284-4155

Mark Mahowald, M.D.
Sleep Disorders Center
Hennepin County Medical
  Center
701 Park Avenue South
Minneapolis, MN 55415
612-347-6288

Jarrett W. Richardson III,
  M.D.
Sleep Disorders Center
Mayo Clinic
200 1st Street, SW
Rochester, MN 55905
507-285-4150

Mark Wedel, M.D.
St. Louis Park
  Medical Center
5000 W. 39th Street
Minneapolis, MN 55416
612-927-3167

Philip R. Westbrook, M.D.
Sleep Disorders Center
Mayo Clinic
200 1st Street, SW
Rochester, MN 55905
507-286-8900

Mississippi

Lawrence S. Schoen, Ph.D.
Sleep Disorders Center
University of Mississippi
  Medical Center
2500 N. State Street
Jackson, MS 39216
601-987-5552

Missouri

Kristyna M. Hartse, Ph.D.
Sleep Disorders Center
St. Louis University
  Medical Center
1221 S. Grand Boulevard
St. Louis, MO 62104
314-771-7600

Paula K. Schweitzer, Ph.D.
Sleep Disorders Center
Deaconess Hospital
6150 Oakland Avenue
St. Louis, MO 63139
314-768-3100

James K. Walsh, Ph.D.
Sleep Disorders Center
Deaconess Hospital
6150 Oakland Avenue
St. Louis, MO 63139
314-768-3100

New Hampshire

Peter J. Hauri, Ph.D.
Sleep Disorders Center
Department of Psychiatry
Dartmouth Medical School
Hanover, NH 03756
603-646-7534

J. Gila Lindsley, Ph.D.
Sleep-Wake Disorders
  Center
Hampstead Hospital
East Road
Hampstead, NH 03841
603-329-5311

Michael J. Sateia, M.D.
Dartmouth-Hitchcock Sleep
  Disorders Center
Department of Psychiatry
Dartmouth Medical School
Hanover, NH 03756
603-646-7534

New Mexico

Wolfgang W. Schmidt-
  Nowara, M.D.
Department of Medicine
Pulmonary Division 7-
  South
University of New Mexico
  Hospital
Albuquerque, NM 87131
505-843-2241

New York

Theodore L. Baker, Ph.D.
Sleep Disorders Center
State University of New
    York at Stony Brook
Stony Brook, NY 11794
516-444-1366

Neil B. Kavey, M.D.
Sleep Disorders Center
Columbia-Presbyterian
    Medical Center
161 Fort Washington
    Avenue
New York, NY 10032
212-694-6100

Charles Pollak, M.D.
Sleep-Wake Disorders Center
New York Hospital–Cornell
    Medical Center
21 Bloomingdale Road
White Plains, NY 10605
914-997-5751

Arthur J. Spielman, Ph.D.
Sleep Disorders Center
City College of New York
New York, NY 10031
212-690-5396

Michael J. Thorpy, M.D.
Sleep-Wake Disorders
    Center
Montefiore Hospital
111 E. 210th Street
Bronx, NY 10467
212-920-4841

Daniel Wagner, M.D.
Sleep-Wake Disorders Center
New York Hospital–Cornell
    Medical Center
21 Bloomingdale Road
White Plains, NY 10605
914-997-5751

North Carolina

Dennis L. Hill, M.D.
Charlotte Neurological
    Clinic
1900 Brunswick Avenue
Charlotte, NC 28207
704-377-9323

Ohio

Robert W. Clark, M.D.
1450 Hawthorne Avenue
Columbus, Ohio 43203
614-258-8466

Dudley S. Dinner, M.D.
Department of Neurology
Cleveland Clinic
9500 Euclid Avenue
Cleveland, OH 44106
216-444-8732

Massimo De Marchis,
    Psy.D.
Kettering Medical Center
3535 Southern Boulevard
Kettering, OH 45429
513-296-7805

Martin B. Scharf, Ph.D.
Cincinnati Sleep Disorders
    Center
515 Melish Avenue
Cincinnati, OH 45229
513-861-7770

Helmut S. Schmidt, M.D.
Ohio State University
    Medical Center
473 W. 12th Avenue
Columbus, OH 43210
614-421-8296

Oklahoma

William C. Orr, Ph.D.
Sleep Disorders Center
Presbyterian Hospital
13th and Lincoln
    Boulevard
Oklahoma City, OK 73104
405-271-6312

Oregon

Gerald B. Rich, M.D.
Neurological Sciences
    Center
Good Samaritan Hospital
2222 N.W. Lovejoy Street
Suite 515
Portland, OR 97210
503-229-7711

Pennsylvania

David Kupfer, M.D.
Sleep Disorders Center
Western Psychiatric
    Institute
3811 O'Hara Street
Pittsburgh, PA 15213
412-624-2246

Mark R. Pressman, Ph.D.
Sleep Disorders Center
Medical College of
    Pennsylvania
330 Henry Avenue
Philadelphia, PA 19129
215-842-4250

Charles F. Reynolds, M.D.
Sleep Disorders Center
Western Psychiatric
    Institute
3811 O'Hara Street
Pittsburgh, PA 15213
412-624-2246

Calvin Stafford, M.D.
Sleep Disorders Center
Crozer-Chester Medical
    Center
Chester, PA 19013
215-447-7688

Rhode Island

Mary A. Carskadon, Ph.D.
Sleep Laboratory
Department of Psychiatry
Bradley Hospital
1011 Veterans Memorial
    Parkway
East Providence, RI 02915
401-434-3400

A. R. Hamel, Ph.D.
203 Governor Street
Providence, RI 02906
401-751-5575

Tennessee

Michael L. Eisenstadt,
   M.D.
930 Emerald Avenue
Suite 815
Knoxville, TN 37917
615-971-6011

J. Brevard Haynes, M.D.
4230 Harding Road
Suite 311
Nashville, TN 37205
615-385-1946

Helio Lemmi, M.D.
899 Madison Avenue
Memphis, TN 38146
901-522-5651

Texas

Barbara J. Beckham, Ph.D.
Sleep/Wake Disorders
   Center
Presbyterian Hospital of
   Dallas
8200 Walnut Hill Lane
Dallas, TX 75231
214-696-8563

Sabri Derman, M.D.
Humana Sleep Disorders
   Center
1303 McCullough Avenue
Suite 447
San Antonio, TX 78212
512-223-4057

Milton K. Erman, M.D.
Sleep/Wake Disorders
   Center
Presbyterian Hospital of
   Dallas
8200 Walnut Hill Lane
Dallas, TX 75231
214-696-8563

John H. Herman, Ph.D.
Department of Psychiatry
University of Texas
   Health Science Center
5323 Harry Hines Boulevard
Dallas, TX 75235
214-688-3040

Ismet Karacan, M.D.
Sleep Disorders Center
Department of Psychiatry
Baylor College of Medicine
Houston, TX 77030
713-790-4886

Ed Lucas, Ph.D.
PO Box 31
Fort Worth, TX 76101
817-926-2544

Howard P. Roffwarg, M.D.
Department of Psychiatry
University of Texas
   Health Science Center
5323 Harry Hines Boulevard
Dallas, TX 75235
214-688-3040

Utah

John M. Andrews, M.D.
Sleep Disorders Center
Utah Neurological Clinic
1999 N. Columbia Lane
Provo, UT 84601
801-226-2300

Virginia

Larry A. Isrow, M.D.
2226 Park Avenue
Richmond, VA 23220
804-786-9349

J. Catesby Ware, Ph.D.
Sleep Disorders Center
Norfolk General Hospital
600 Gresham Drive
Norfolk, VA 23507
804-628-3322

Wisconsin

Steven Weber, Ph.D.
Milwaukee Sleep Disorders
  Center
Columbia Hospital
2025 E. Newport Avenue
Milwaukee, WI 53211
414-961-4650

CANADA

Roger Broughton, M.D.
Division of Neurology
Ottawa General Hospital
Room LM-15
Ottawa, Ontario, Canada
  K1H 8L6
613-737-8155

Alan B. Douglass, M.D.
University of Alberta
1-134 Clinical Sciences
  Building
Edmonton, Alberta, Canada
  T6G 2G3
403-432-6578

Index

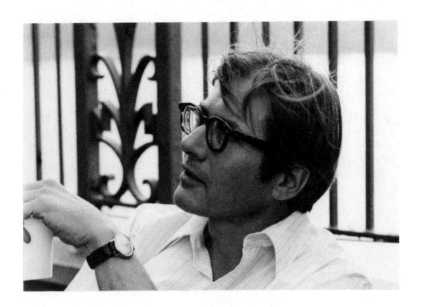

About the Author

Ernest Hartmann is a well-known pioneer in research on sleep and sleep disorders whose work also includes teaching and maintaining a private practice in sleep disorders medicine and psychiatry. It is only during the past thirty years or so that sleep has been seriously studied by scientists, and Dr. Hartmann has been in the field for twenty-five of these years. He is currently professor of psychiatry at Tufts University School of Medicine, director of the Sleep Research Laboratory of West-Ros-Park Mental Health Center at Lemuel Shattuck Hospital, and director of the Sleep Disorders Center of the Newton-Wellesley Hospital, 2014 Washington Street, Newton, Massachusetts 02162, (617) 243-6624. He is medical director of the Sleep Research Foundation.

Born in Vienna, Austria, Dr. Hartmann went to high school in New York, received his undergraduate degree from the University of Chicago, received his medical degree from the Yale University School of Medicine, and is a graduate of the Boston Psychoanalytic Institute and a member of its faculty.

Dr. Hartmann is the author of four previous books on sleep and dreaming—including the widely quoted *The Nightmare: The Biology and Psychology of Terrifying Dreams*—and the editor of another and has published over 250 scientific articles. He lives in Newton, Massachusetts, with his wife, Eva, and has two children.

Information You Can Count On!

821. **239 Ways to Put Your Money to Work.** $8.95 / AARP member price $6.50.

822. **Sunbelt Retirement:** The Complete State-by-State Guide. $11.95 / AARP member price $8.50.

824. **Walking for the Health of It.** The Easy and Effective Exercise for People Over 50. $6.95 / AARP member price $4.95.

826. **Think of Your Future.** Preretirement Planning Workbook. $24.95 / AARP member price $18.25.

829. **Retirement Edens Outside the Sunbelt.** $10.95 / AARP member price $7.95.

With more than 25 million members, the American Association of Retired Persons is the world's largest membership and service organization for people over 50 and the leading authority on matters of interest to them. That knowledge and authority stand behind every AARP book.

HOW TO ORDER

To order state book name and number, quantity and price (AARP members: be sure to include your membership no. for discount) and add $1.75 *per entire order* for shipping and handling. *All orders must be prepaid.* For your convenience we accept checks, money orders, VISA and MasterCard (credit card orders must include card no., exp. date and cardholder signature). *Please allow 4 weeks for delivery.*

Send your order today to:

AARP Books / Scott, Foresman and Co., 1865 Miner Street Des Plaines, IL 60016

AARP Books are co-published by AARP and Scott, Foresman and Co., sold by Scott, Foresman a Co., and distributed to bookstores by Farrar, Straus and Giroux.

Join AARP today and enjoy valuable benefits

65% of dues is designated for Association publications. Dues outside continental U.S.: $7 one year, $18 three years. Please allow 3 to 6 weeks for receipt of membership kit.

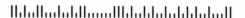